O A N L
OXFORD AMERICAN NEUROLOGY LIBRARY

Alzheimer's Disease and Its Variants: A Diagnostic and Therapeutic Guide

This material is not intended to be, and should not be considered, a substitute for medical or other professional advice. Treatment for the conditions described in this material is highly dependent on the individual circumstances. While this material is designed to offer accurate information with respect to the subject matter covered and to be current as of the time it was written, research and knowledge about medical and health issues are constantly evolving, and dose schedules for medications are being revised continually, with new side effects recognized and accounted for regularly. Readers must therefore always check the product information and clinical procedures with the most up-to-date published product information and data sheets provided by the manufacturers and the most recent codes of conduct and safety regulation. Oxford University Press and the authors make no representations or warranties to readers, express or implied, as to the accuracy or completeness of this material, including without limitation that they make no representations or warranties as to the accuracy or efficacy of the drug dosages mentioned in the material. The authors and the publishers do not accept, and expressly disclaim, any responsibility for any liability, loss, or risk that may be claimed or incurred as a consequence of the use and/or application of any of the contents of this material.

The Publisher is responsible for author selection and the Publisher and the Author(s) make all editorial decisions, including decisions regarding content. The Publisher and the Author(s) are not responsible for any product information added to this publication by companies purchasing copies of it for distribution to clinicians.

O A N L
OXFORD AMERICAN NEUROLOGY LIBRARY

Alzheimer's Disease and Its Variants: A Diagnostic and Therapeutic Guide

Richard J. Caselli, MD

Professor and Chair,
Department of Neurology,
Mayo Clinic, Arizona

Clinical Core Director,
Arizona Alzheimer's Disease Center

Pierre N. Tariot, MD

Director,
Banner Alzheimer's Institute Memory Disorders Center

Research Professor,
Psychiatry, University of Arizona College of Medicine

OXFORD
UNIVERSITY PRESS

2010

OXFORD
UNIVERSITY PRESS

Oxford University Press, Inc., publishes works that further
Oxford University's objective of excellence
in research, scholarship, and education.

Oxford New York

Auckland Cape Town Dar es Salaam Hong Kong Karachi
Kuala Lumpur Madrid Melbourne Mexico City Nairobi
New Delhi Shanghai Taipei Toronto

With offices in
Argentina Austria Brazil Chile Czech Republic France Greece
Guatemala Hungary Italy Japan Poland Portugal Singapore
South Korea Switzerland Thailand Turkey Ukraine Vietnam

Copyright © 2010 by Oxford University Press, Inc.

Published by Oxford University Press, Inc.
198 Madison Avenue, New York, New York 10016
www.oup.com

Oxford is a registered trademark of Oxford University Press

Library of Congress Cataloging-in-Publication Data

Caselli, Richard J.
Alzheimer's disease and its variants : a diagnostic and therapeutic guide / Richard J.
Caselli, Pierre N. Tariot.
    p. ; cm. — (Oxford American neurology library)
Includes bibliographical references and index.
ISBN 978-0-19-539338-5 (standard ed. : alk. paper)   1. Alzheimer's disease.
2. Dementia.   I. Tariot, Pierre N.   II. Title.   III. Series: Oxford American
neurology library.
[DNLM: 1. Alzheimer Disease—diagnosis. 2. Alzheimer Disease—therapy. 3. Dementia—
diagnosis. 4. Dementia—therapy. 5. Long-Term Care. WT 155 C337a 2010]
RC523.C383 2010
616.8′31—dc22   2009022266

Printed in the United States of America
on acid-free paper

Acknowledgments

We are witnessing a "perfect storm" of converging medical, social, and economic calamities that threaten to undermine the already challenged U.S. healthcare system, and Alzheimer's disease may be its focal point. Our aging baby boomers are driving up the numbers of people who suffer and will suffer from this still incurable chronic disabling disease just as medical reimbursement for the care of these individuals falls to an all-time low. The number of healthcare professionals needed to confront this challenge far outpaces the number who are entering the specialties of behavioral neurology, geriatric psychiatry, and geriatric medicine. Remaining on the front lines of the healthcare delivery war are primary care physicians and a relatively new but rapidly growing breed of healthcare professional, the midlevel provider (nurse practitioners and physician assistants). These are the soldiers who will confront the swell of dementia patients, and it is to these professionals that we dedicate and focus this book. We intend this book to be a field manual for such providers for the diagnosis and treatment of Alzheimer's disease in all its forms.

In designing this book, we have deliberately emphasized treatment. Because Alzheimer's disease is not yet curable, it must be managed for a long period of time. The types of management challenges that arise are many, but often predictable. Diagnosis is often the key to management as symptoms determine needs that in turn determine interventions. The mind is like a house with many rooms in it. Memory is one of those rooms, but it is not the whole house. We have used this analogy to demystify cognitive diagnosis. There are office-based tools that are brief and simple that can be used to paint a picture of a cognitive syndrome, thus aiding clinical diagnosis. Alzheimer's disease is Alzheimer's disease first and foremost because it looks like Alzheimer's disease. It is not simply a diagnosis of exclusion. This approach will allow nonspecialists to learn to see what Alzheimer's disease and all its variant forms looks like, thus providing greater certainty about diagnosis and treatment.

We have been exceptionally fortunate to receive the help of some extraordinary people who we wish to publicly acknowledge. Geri R. Hall, PhD, CNP, contributed to our chapters on nonpharmacological management. Her expertise in this area is legendary and we hope our readers will benefit as much as we and our patients have. Jan Dougherty, RN, MS, contributed her considerable expertise on end-of-life care in patients with dementia that she implements daily in a unique comprehensive dementia-care program she and Geri Hall helped to design. John Hardy, PhD, genetics pioneer, visionary, and author of the amyloid cascade hypothesis, the reigning paradigm of Alzheimer's disease pathogenesis, provided a review of the early manuscript, as well as an updated figure of the amyloid cascade hypothesis. For all his encouragement, support, and friendship over the years we are very grateful. Eric M. Reiman, MD, our collaborative partner in research and dear friend, has been ever supportive and contributed some amazing radiological images, including amyloid imaging in presymptomatic individuals at risk for Alzheimer's disease. Tom Beach, MD, has kept our clinical acumens sharp with his neuropathological insights and correlations in patients we have seen. He is a wonderful and patient teacher, and both he and our colleague Dr. Dennis Dickson generously contributed photomicrographs of the neuropathological substrates that define Alzheimer's disease. Mr. Thomas Bibby patiently worked with Dr. Caselli creating the "houses of the mind" that we hope will demystify cognitive examination and diagnosis.

Finally, we wish to thank our patients and our colleagues with whom we work every day. Our goals are to maintain the quality of life and dignity of patients and families affected by Alzheimer's disease and all forms of dementia, and to advance our understanding of this disease in the hope that one day our work will contribute to a cure. But until there is a cure, our patients and families have a lot of life left to live, and we hope this book will help those who are trying to help them live that life well.

Contents

Section E: Experimental and future therapies
P.N. Tariot

Section A

The diagnosis and evaluation of dementia

The term "dementia" has an intellectually constricting effect on clinicians. Some have even argued the term is frankly offensive (1). This may seem an odd way to introduce a book on Alzheimer's disease, but until there is a cure or highly effective therapy, a patient's greatest hope lies in the active consideration of alternative diagnoses with greater therapeutic potential. For example, a confused elderly person seen for the first time might appear to be "demented" but may actually be experiencing a reversible delirium induced by sepsis or medication toxicity. Further, even patients with established dementia due to Alzheimer's disease (AD) or any other cause may experience abrupt deterioration that itself may reflect a potentially reversible, nondegenerative exacerbating factor. When confronted by such patients we must, therefore, be vigilant and our approach to such patients thorough and definitive.

With the graying of our population, the oldest old are the most rapidly growing demographic. The number of patients with AD and related forms of dementia will continue to balloon, and primary care will be the front line of our medical defenses. There will not be enough specialists to manage all of these patients, and so it is to our front-line healthcare providers that we dedicate this book. Our goal is to provide practical diagnostic and therapeutic information so that this might serve as a "battlefield manual" for dementia management. Although the book is about AD, the principles it describes apply to all forms of dementia. We hope it will serve you well.

References

1. Trachtenberg DI, Trojanowski JQ. Dementia: a word to be forgotten. Arch Neurol 2008;65(5):593–595.

Chapter 1

Normal aging and memory decline

Cognitive Aging and the Risk of Alzheimer's Disease

Alzheimer's disease (AD) is common and becoming more so. The estimated number of Americans with Alzheimer's disease has doubled since 1980 to 4.5 million, and is expected to triple again by 2050 (1). Our population is aging, and age, the strongest risk factor for developing AD, accounts for the vast majority of cases. The public is highly aware of AD, making it a major health-related concern of aging patients and their families (2), who consequently express concern about memory lapses and related cognitive errors to their physicians at increasingly earlier disease stages. This raises a common diagnostic conundrum: when does normal cognitive aging become pathological cognitive decline?

Cognitive profiles of normal aging emphasize declining learning efficiency (how many learning trials needed to remember something), working memory (holding something in "the mind's eye" while working on it, such as repeating a string of numbers backwards; or multitasking, considering multiple things at once), and psychomotor speed (how quickly it takes to do something such as reciting all the words that begin with the letter "C") (3–5); all these are thought to reflect impairment of frontal lobe function (Fig. 1.1). Memory loss, as the term is generally used by patients, family members, and most physicians, refers to impaired delayed recall of previously learned or previously known information. It is thought to reflect impairment of medial temporal lobe and possibly basal forebrain function, and is generally the earliest cognitive change caused by AD (6–11) (Fig. 1.1).

These cognitive profiles overlap, however, so that distinguishing normal aging from early-stage AD can be difficult (12,13) (Fig. 1.1).

Insights into the distinction between the two that may be helpful for counseling worried patients and family members have been gained from studies of healthy-appearing people at predictably different levels of risk for the future development of AD. The apolipoprotein E (APOE) e4 allele is the most prevalent known genetic risk factor for AD and perhaps the second most important risk factor (after aging) overall. Roughly 20% to 25% of people in North America and Europe have at least one copy of this gene, and it is estimated to account for as many as half of all sporadic and familial late-onset cases (14,15). APOE e4-related AD age of onset is typically after age 65 years, although rarely APOE e4 may be a genetic cause of dementia prior to age 60 (16). Longitudinal observational studies have shown that healthy-appearing APOE e4 carriers in their 50s and 60s experience more rapidly progressive age-related declines in learning efficiency and memory than age-matched matched APOE e4 noncarriers (17–19). Whether such accelerated decline increases age-related memory complaints in e4 carriers, however, remains uncertain. The e4 effect is detectable as a difference between large groups, but at the individual level, it remains very difficult to disambiguate from normal forgetfulness (Fig. 1.2).

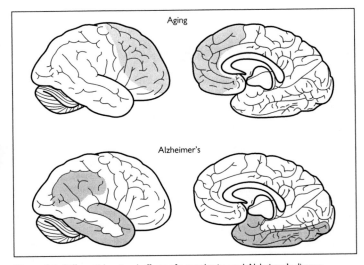

Figure 1.1 Differential regional effects of normal aging and Alzheimer's disease.

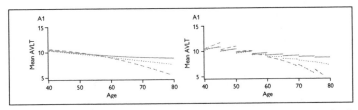

Figure 1.2 Memory declines with age in APOE genetic subgroups (e4 noncarriers [top], heterozygotes [middle] and homozygotes [bottom]) even in the absence of clinically symptomatic Alzheimer's disease. A1 depicts baseline differences in memory performance with age, while A2 depicts longitudinal change in performance. Memory decline is greatest in APOE e4 homozygotes, and least in e4 noncarriers.

Reprinted with permission from Caselli RJ, Dueck AC, Osborne D, Sabbagh MN, Connor DJ, Ahern GL, Baxter LC, Rapcsak SZ, Shi J, Woodruff BK, Locke DE, Snyder CH, Alexander GE, Rademakers R, Reiman EM. Longitudinal modeling of age-related memory decline and the APOE epsilon4 effect. N Engl J Med 2009 Jul 16; 361(3):255–63.

Objectively, however, such decline correlates with reduced cerebral metabolism on fluorodeoxyglucose (FDG) positron emission tomography (PET) scans (suggesting it may reflect early-stage AD) as much as 5 to 10 years before the onset of cognitive symptoms (20) (Fig. 1.3).

Regarding the concerns of patients under the age of 50, the literature is divided on the potential effect of APOE e4 on cognitive functioning in healthy younger adults. In the religious order study by Snowdon, psycholinguistic differences in 20-year-old women correlated with AD and neuropathological disease burden 60 years later (21). Whalley et al found that school-age performances on psychometric tests in a cohort of Scottish children were predictive of dementia by the time these children reached old age (22). In contrast, Caselli et al found no correlation between APOE genotype and intellectual achievement as measured by educational and occupational outcomes (23), although middle-aged APOE e4 homozygotes may be more sensitive to the effects of fatigue (24) and anxiety (25) than e4 noncarriers. Most data suggest that age-related cognitive decline prior to age 50 is essentially identical in e4 carriers and noncarriers as a group, and any childhood or young adult differences are likely to be lifelong and superimposed on this APOE–age interaction (whether or not such differences might predispose to the subsequent development of dementia).

In summary, mild memory decline occurs as a normal accompaniment of aging, but memory declines more steeply with advancing age in those at greater genetic risk for AD. Group-level analyses can make these differences seem obvious, but the clinician's task of distinguishing such a difference in an individual patient remains much more challenging and requires a careful diagnostic evaluation.

Factors Influencing Self- and Observer-Perceived Cognitive Loss

Because the perception of cognitive impairment is at least partially subjective, we must understand what influences the perception and reporting of cognitive loss by the patient and by observers so that we may better judge when reported cognitive loss is truly a cause for concern.

Let us begin with a patient who seems reasonably intact, perhaps even a colleague, who is expressing concern about his or her memory (e.g., "I had trouble finding my car in the staff parking lot"). There is no history of impaired work performance, and on formal examination he or she has no apparent cognitive or neurological deficits. Why does this person perceive that he or she has memory loss? There are several possible reasons.

First, there is indeed something neurologically wrong, but it is subtle and escaping detection by our office-based assessment. This could reflect the patient's educational and language background. High-functioning people can often "pass" mental status tests during the early stages of AD yet correctly self-perceive they have a problem. Conversely, errors made by patients with low

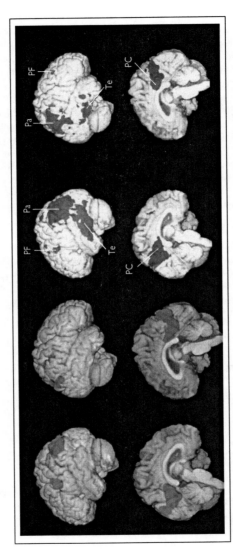

Figure 1.3 FDG PET of healthy APOE e4 carriers (left) and Alzheimer's disease patients (right) demonstrating similar but less extensive reduction in cerebral metabolism in presymptomatic e4 carriers. This is not the distribution of maximum neuropathology, and the reason for this characteristic pattern is debated. PF = Prefrontal, Pa = Parietal, Te = Temporal, PC = Posterior Cingulate. (Figures courtesy of Dr. Eric M. Reiman)

educational backgrounds or those who are tested in a language in which they normally struggle can be "forgiven" too much and their errors assumed to reflect nonmedical factors. Another possibility regards the nature of the impairment. A variety of cognitive syndromes that are caused by variants of AD and other disorders can begin with language, movement, visuospatial, or executive difficulties. Most office-based mental status tests emphasize memory loss as a marker for early cognitive impairment, and so mild forms of nonamnestic syndromes are easily missed in the absence of formal neuropsychological assessment.

A second possibility is that there is no strictly neurological problem, but the patient is systemically ill and experiencing secondary cognitive symptoms. Consider that we prefer not to take the SATs or MCATs when we have the flu. Fatigue (which itself can result from sleep apnea or a myriad of other causes), depression, medications, and a variety of systemic medical problems can secondarily affect the efficiency of our cognitive skills in nonspecific but organic ways (26,27). It is therefore important to determine what the patient is actually describing, and specific examples of the problem can be helpful to ascertain this.

Third, studies have shown that the strongest correlate of cognitive complaints is emotional distress (28,29). In other words, anxiety and depression account for more cognitive complaints than AD or related cognitive disorders. This affects not only patients themselves but also spouses, children, friends, and other observers. "Either he is developing dementia or else he is an inconsiderate S.O.B." are words we have heard from several patients' spouses (in one case we obtained autopsy proof that the patient had no degenerative brain disease, although we would not consider that neuropathological proof of the spouse's other diagnostic consideration!).

Fourth, the patient may be right, despite normal examination findings. As illustrated, there is a great deal of historical "noise," but some individuals with early cognitive decline accurately report that they perceive themselves to be cognitively struggling, a perception that longitudinal follow-up confirms, even in the absence of impaired cross-sectional psychometric performance at the baseline evaluation. It is the element of change that is critical. It is less concerning to hear that a patient has always had a bad memory than to hear that his memory is getting worse "and these are some concrete examples that show why I think so," especially if confirmed by a corroborating historian. While difficult to demonstrate, longitudinal studies have shown that objective neuropsychological decline, especially in a cognitive domain–specific pattern (i.e., multiple tests within a specific cognitive domain such as memory, language, spatial, or executive skills), correlates with genetic risk for AD and precedes symptomatic AD by several years (19).

Even in patients with frank dementia, there are multiple issues that affect self- and observer-based perceptions of cognitive functioning. The first step in any medical evaluation is to take a history. When the evaluation of cognitive impairment must account for the possibility of AD, there are several potentially confounding factors to consider. First, patients who really have impaired memory can fail to recall salient details of their problem. Second, some patients with AD have anosognosia, the denial of illness. The solution is a corroborating historian, such as a spouse. It is still appropriate to begin the history by asking the patient what he or she feels is wrong, but it is imperative to then obtain the corroborating historian's version of the history. A further potentially confounding factor, however, is a reluctant or fearful corroborating historian. Some simply do not want to hurt their loved one's feelings, while others may be frankly afraid, especially if the patient has become paranoid or belligerent (as can result from AD). In this case, it is important to provide the corroborating historian with a confidential communication avenue such as interviewing him or her separately, or writing a letter describing the problem.

Circumstance may affect our perception of disease course, a diagnostically important detail in the evaluation of AD. While AD is a gradually progressive problem, occasionally family members will perceive and report the abrupt onset of symptoms. Usually the reason reflects either something about the observer, the situation, or a concurrent problem. For example, a daughter comes home for a holiday and is surprised by the change she sees in her father. No such change was previously noted by the mother, but with certain changes called to her attention, she agrees that the father was not like this before. Alternatively, a patient may be coping with his simple, quiet life until left alone in a crowded airport, where he becomes lost, or at the holidays, when two dozen guests arrive, with resulting cacophony and perhaps some alcohol. Or, a seemingly normal elderly patient develops delirium after heart surgery; it never seems to completely clear and is followed by ongoing decline. In each case, subtle decline had likely been occurring even before the observer or circumstance changed.

In summary, multiple factors influence the perception and reporting of cognitive decline by patients and their families. In patients whose office examination seems normal, formal medical and neuropsychological evaluations are appropriate to more sensitively identify an underlying cognitive or medical disorder and can establish a baseline against which to judge future performance. Even in patients with frank dementia, AD itself can alter a person's self-perception, and a patient's behavioral changes can influence how a spouse chooses to report his or her observations.

Risk Factors for Dementia

AD is the most common cause of dementia, accounting for more than half of all cases. Other common causes include vascular dementia and dementia with Lewy bodies, both of which are often accompanied pathologically by AD. Frontotemporal lobar degeneration (that includes Pick's disease) is less common but can be mimicked by AD. Even repetitive head injury, a cause of dementia typically occurring in boxers (dementia pugilistica), is accompanied by AD-like pathology. In all of these cases, age plays an important role, even though there are other important factors in those with a nondegenerative component (vascular dementia and dementia pugilistica), and the usual age of onset is slightly younger in patients with frontotemporal lobar degeneration.

Epidemiological age-specific estimates of incidence and prevalence vary by region (within the United States and globally) and study due to differences in diagnostic criteria and population demographics. There is an exponential increase in both with advancing age at least through the ninth decade (1), and recent evidence suggests this trend continues into the tenth decade (2). The prevalence of severe dementia over the age of 60 is estimated at 5%, and over the age of 85, between 20% and 50%. The lifetime risk of developing AD is estimated to be between 12% and 17% (30,32).

Following age, APOE genetic status is the second most important risk factor.

In both familial late-onset (14) and sporadic (15) cases, the APOE e4 allele increases risk and the e2 allele decreases risk (33). The lifetime risk of AD in people without a family history increases from 9% without an APOE e4 allele to 29% with one copy of the APOE e4 allele (34). APOE e4 homozygotes make

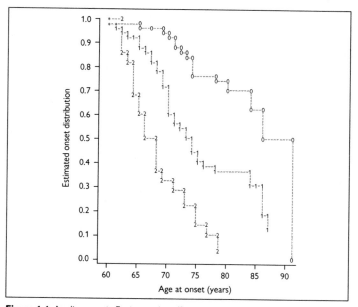

Figure 1.4 Apolipoprotein E e4 gene dose (from top to bottom graph are e4 noncarriers/no copies, e4 heterozygotes/one copy, e4 homozygotes/two copies) shifts the age of onset of Alzheimer's disease younger, and increases the likelihood of onset. From Corder EH, Saunders AM, Strittmatter WJ, et al: Gene dose of apolipoprotein E type 4 allele and the risk of Alzheimer's disease in late onset families. Science 1993;261:921–923 (14). Reprinted with permission from AAAS.

up roughly 2% of the population, but approximately 83% are estimated to develop AD in their lifetime (35), similar to the 91% reported in familial late-onset cases (14,15). The prevalence of the APOE e4 allele varies globally, as does age-adjusted dementia prevalence, so that there is generally a lower prevalence in Mediterranean and Asian countries and a higher prevalence in Northern than in Southern European countries (36–38). Family history of dementia, especially in a first-degree relative, even in the absence of APOE e4 remains a risk factor for AD, and in limited populations, other genetic factors play a determining role, such as Down syndrome (trisomy 21) (39) and autosomal dominant mutation early-onset familial AD kindreds.

Cognitive impairment can also result from stroke, and such impairment can be disabling, thus fulfilling one of the defining characteristics of dementia. Terminology is debated, but atherosclerosis and atherosclerotic risk factors enhance the risk of stroke, vascular cognitive impairment, and vascular (previously termed "multi-infarct") dementia. Given the frequent coexistence of AD in patients with vascular dementia, vascular risk factors that include diabetes mellitus (40), the metabolic syndrome (41), hypercholesterolemia (or some form of related genetic or metabolic effect) (42,43), and intracranial atherosclerosis (44) have also been suggested to enhance the risk of AD, although not all studies have confirmed this (45).

Dream enactment behavior is the cardinal feature of REM sleep behavior disorder (RBD), and whether it is regarded as a risk factor or as an early symptomatic stage of disease, it is associated with the synucleinopathies (degenerative diseases characterized pathologically by neuronal inclusions termed "Lewy bodies" composed of alpha-synuclein) that include Parkinson's disease, dementia with Lewy bodies (which in turn is frequently associated with AD), and multiple system atrophy (46). Individuals who otherwise appear to be neurologically and cognitively healthy who develop RBD are at risk for the further evolution of parkinsonism, dementia, and/or dysautonomia. Although the exact level of risk is not yet clear (47,48), a recent prospective study of 93 patients showed the risk of neurodegenerative disease to be 17.7% in 5 years, 40.6% in 10 years, and 52.4% in 12 years (49). Further, other factors, including post-traumatic stress disorder (50) and certain medications (particularly the selective serotonin reuptake inhibitor antidepressants) (51), predispose to dream enactment behavior, making it less clear whether RBD necessarily results from a neurodegenerative process.

Other purported factors for AD that are less clear-cut but may modestly influence overall risk include education (52), depression (53), head trauma (54), diet (55), intellectual activity (56), and physical exercise (57). Epidemiologic studies (the Women's Health Initiative Memory Study) have cast serious doubt on previously held putative benefits of estrogen replacement therapy (58). Finally, some previously held factors have undergone testing in randomized controlled clinical trials and failed to show any benefit. These include vitamin E (59), vitamins B6, B12, and folic acid (to reduce serum homocysteine) (60), anti-inflammatory drugs (61), and gingko biloba (62).

References

1. Hebert LE, Scherr PA, Bienas JL, et al. Alzheimer disease in the U.S. population: prevalence estimates using the 2000 census. Arch Neurol 2003;60:1119–1122.

2. Caspermeyer JJ, Sylvester EJ, Drazkowski JF, et all. Evaluation of stigmatizing language and medical errors in neurology coverage by US newspapers. Mayo Clin Proc 2006;81(3):300–306.

3. West RL. An application of prefrontal cortex function theory to cognitive aging. Psychol Bull 1996;120:272–292.

4. Verhaeghen P, Cerella J. Aging, executive control, and attention: a review of meta-analyses. Neurosci Behav Rev 2002;26:849–857.

5. Treitz FH, Heyder K, Daum I. Differential course of executive control changes during normal aging. Aging Neuropsychol Cognition 2007;14:370–393.

6. Petersen RC, Smith GE, Waring SC, et al. Mild cognitive impairment: clinical characterization and outcome. Arch Neurol 1999;56:303–308.

7. Morris JC, Storandt M, Miller JP, et al. Mild cognitive impairment represents early stage Alzheimer disease. Arch Neurol 2001;58:397–405.

8. Petersen RC, Stevens JC, Ganguli M, et al. Practice parameter: early detection of dementia: mild cognitive impairment (an evidence-based review). Report of the Quality Standards Subcommittee of the American Academy of Neurology. Neurology 2001;56:1133–1142.

9. Boyle PA, Wilson RS, Aggarwal NT, et al. Mild cognitive impairment: risk of Alzheimer's disease and rate of cognitive decline. Neurology 2006;67:441–445.

10. Albert M, Blacker D, Moss MB, et al. Longitudinal change in cognitive performance among individuals with mild cognitive impairment. Neuropsychology 2007;21:158–169.

11. Howieson DB, Carlson NE, Moore MM, et al. Trajectory of mild cognitive impairment onset. J Int Neuropsychol Soc 2008;14:192–198.

12. Salthouse TA. Memory aging 18 to 80. Alzeimer Dis Assoc Disord 2003;17: 162–167.

13. Burke D, Mackay DG. Memory, language, and ageing. Phil Trans R Soc Lond B 1997;352:1845–1856.

14. Corder EH, Saunders AM, Strittmatter WJ, et al. Gene dose of apoipoprotein E type 4 allele and the risk of AD in late onset families. Science 1993;261(5123):921–923.

15. Saunders AM, Strittmatter WJ, Schmechel D, et al. Association of apolipoprotein E allele ε4 with late onset familial and sporadic Alzheimer's disease. Neurology 1993;43:1467–1472.

16. Brickell KL, Steinbart EJ, Rumbaugh M, et al. Early-onset Alzheimer disease families with late-onset Alzheimer disease: a potential important subtype of familial Alzheimer disease. Arch Neurol 2006;63:1307–1311.

17. Baxter LC, Caselli RJ, Johnson SC, et al. Apolipoprotein E epsilon 4 affects new learning in cognitively normal individuals at risk for Alzheimer's disease. Neurobiol Aging 2003;24(7):947–952.

18. Caselli RJ, Reiman EM, Osborne D, et al. Longitudinal changes in cognition and behavior in asymptomatic carriers of the APOE e4 allele. Neurology 2004;62(11):1990–1995.

19. Caselli RJ, Reiman EM, Locke DE, et al. Cognitive domain decline in healthy apolipoprotein E epsilon4 homozygotes before the diagnosis of mild cognitive impairment. Arch Neurol 2007;64(9):1306–1311.

20. Caselli RJ, Chen K, Lee W, et al. Correlating cerebral hypometabolism with future memory decline in subsequent converters to amnestic pre-mild cognitive impairment. Arch Neurol 2008;65:1231–1236.

21. Snowden DA. Healthy aging and dementia: findings from the nun study. Ann Intern Med 2003;139:450–454.

22. Whalley LJ, Starr JM, Athawes R, et al. Childhood mental ability and dementia. Neurology 2000;55:1455–1459.

23. Caselli RJ, Hentz JG, Osborne D, et al. Apolipoprotein E and intellectual achievement. J Am Geriatr Soc 2002;50:49–54.

24. Caselli RJ, Reiman EM, Hentz JG, et al. A distinctive interaction between memory and chronic daytime somnolence in asymptomatic APOE e4 homozygotes. Sleep 2002;25:447–453.

25. Caselli RJ, Reiman EM, Hentz JG, et al. A distinctive interaction between chronic anxiety and problem solving in asymptomatic APOE e4 homozygotes. J Neuropsychiatry Clin Neurosci 2004;16:320–329.

26. Haimov I, Hanuka E, Horowitz Y. Chronic insomnia and cognitive functioning among older adults. Behav Sleep Med 2008;6(1):32–54.

27. Caselli RJ. Obstructive sleep apnea, apolipoprotein E e4, and mild cognitive impairment. Sleep Med 2008;9(8):816–817.

28. Weaver Cargin J, Collie A, Masters C, et al. The nature of cognitive complaints in healthy older adults with and without objective memory decline. J Clin Exp Neuropsychol 2008;30(2):245–257.

29. Mitchell AJ. Is it time to separate subjective cognitive complaints from the diagnosis of mild cognitive impairment? Age Ageing 2008;37(5):497–499.

30. Kokmen E, Beard CM, O'Brien PC, et al. Epidemiology of dementia in Rochester, Minnesota. Mayo Clin Proc 1996;71:275–282.

31. Corrada MM, Brookmeyer R, Berlau D, et al. Prevalence of dementia after age 90: results from the 90+ study. Neurology 2008;71:337–343.

32. Farrer LA, Cupples LA. Estimating the probability for major gene Alzheimer disease. Am J Hum Genet 1994;54:374–383.

33. Corder EH, Saunders AM, Risch NJ, et al. Protective effect of apolipoprotein E type 2 allele for late onset Alzheimer disease. Nat Genet 1994;7:180–184.

34. Seshadri S, Drachman DA, Lippa CF. Apolipoprotein E e4 allele and the lifetime risk of Alzheimer's disease. Arch Neurol 1995;52:1074–1079.

35. Poirer J, Davignon D, Bouthillier D, et al. Apolipoprotein E polymorphism and Alzheimer's disease. Lancet 1993;ii:697–699.

36. Gerdes LU, Klausen IC, Sihm I, et al. Apolipoprotein E polymorphism in a Danish population compared to findings in 45 other study populations around the world. Genet Epidemiol 1992;9:155–167.

37. Corbo RM, Scacchi R. Apolipoprotein E (APOE) allele distribution in the world: is APOE4 a "thrifty" allele? Am Hum Genet 1999;63:301–310.

38. Zekraoui L, LaGarde JP, Raisonnier A, et al. High frequency of the apolipoprotein E4 allele in African Pygmies and most of the African Sub-Saharan populations in Sub-Saharan Africa. Hum Biol 1997;69:575–581.

39. Wisniewski KE, Wisniewski HM, Wen GY. Occurrence of neuropathological changes and dementia of Alzheimer's disease in Down's syndrome. Ann Neurol 1985;17:278–282.

40. Ott A, Stolk RP, van Harskamp F, et al. Diabetes mellitus and the risk of dementia: the Rotterdam study. Neurology 1999;53:1937–1942.

41. Vanhanen M, Koivisto K, Moilanen L, et al. Association of metabolic syndrome with Alzheimer disease: a population-based study. Neurology 2006;67:843–847.

42. Wang B, Zhang C, Zheng W, et al. Association between a T/C polymorphism in intron 2 of cholesterol 24S-hydroxylase gene and Alzheimer's disease in Chinese. Neurosci Lett 2004;369:104–107.

43. Papassotiropoulos A, Fountoulakis M, Dunckley T, et al. Genetics, transcriptomics, and proteomics of Alzheimer's disease. J Clin Psychiatry 2006;67:652–670.

44. Roher AE, Esh C, Rahman A, et al. Atherosclerosis of cerebral arteries in Alzheimer disease. Stroke 2004;35:2623–2627.

45. Schneider JA, Wilson RS, Bienias JL, et al. Cerebral infarctions and the likelihood of dementia from Alzheimer disease pathology. Neurology 2004;62:1148–1155.

46. Goedert M. Alpha-synuclein and neurodegerative diseases. Nat Rev Neurosci 2001;2:492–501.

47. Schenck CH, Bunlie SR, Mahowald MW. Delayed emergence of a parkinsonian disorder in 38% of 29 older men initially diagnosed with idiopathic rapid eye movement sleep behavior disorder. Neurology 1996;46:388–393.

48. Caselli RJ, Chen K, Bandy D, et al. A preliminary fluorodeoxyglucose positron emission tomography study in healthy adults reporting dream-enactment behavior. Sleep 2006;29(7):927–933.

49. Postuma RB, Gagnon JF, Vendette M, et al. Quantifying the risk of neurodegenerative disease in idiopathic REM sleep behavior disorder. Neurology 2009;72:1296–1300.

50. Husain AM, Miller PP, Carwile ST. REM sleep behavior disorder: potential relationship to post-traumatic stress disorder. J Clin Neurophysiol 2001;18:148–157.

51. Winkelman JW, James L. Serotonergic antidepressants are associated with REM sleep without atonia. Sleep 2004;27:317–321.

52. Stern Y, Gurland B, Tatemichi TK, et al. Influence of education and occupation on the incidence of Alzheimer's disease. JAMA 1974;271:1004–1010.

53. Chen R, Hu Z, Wei L, et al. Severity of depression and risk for subsequent dementia: cohort studies in China and the UK. Br J Psychiatry 2008;193:373–377.

54. Schofield PW, Tang M, Marder K, et al. Alzheimer's disease after remote head injury: an incidence study. Arch Neurol 1997;62:119–124.

55. Scarmeas N, Stern Y, Tang MX, et al. Mediterranean diet and risk for Alzheimer's disease. Ann Neurol 2006;59:912–921.

56. Wilson RS, Mendes De Leon CF, Barnes LL, et al. Pain cognitively stimulating activities and risk of incident Alzheimer disease. JAMA 2002;287:742–748.

57. Ravaglia G, Forti P, Lucicesare A, et al. Physical activity and dementia risk in the elderly: findings from a prospective Italian study. Neurology 2008;70:1786–1794.

58. Shumaker SA, Legault C, Thal, L, et al. Estrogen plus progestin and the incidence of dementia and mild cognitive impairment in postmenopausal women: the Women's Health Initiative Memory Study, a randomized controlled trial. JAMA 2003;289:2651–2662.

59. Petersen RC, Thomas RG, Grundman M, et al. Vitamin E and donepezil for the treatment of mild cognitive impairment. N Engl J Med 2005;352:2379–2388.

60. Aisen PS, Schneider LS, Sano M, et al. High-dose B vitamin supplementation and cognitive decline in Alzheimer disease: a randomized controlled trial. JAMA 2008;300:1774–1783.

61. Aisen PS, Schafer KA, Grundman M, et al. Effects of rofecoxib or naproxen vs placebo on Alzheimer disease progression: a randomized controlled trial. JAMA 2003;289:2819–2826.

62. DeKosky ST, Williamson JD, Fitzpatrick AL, et al. Gingko biloba for prevention of dementia: a randomized controlled trial. JAMA 2008;300:2253–2262.

Chapter 2

Characterizing a cognitive disorder

Cognitive Domains: Amnesia, Aphasia, Apraxia, Agnosia, Psychomotor Slowing, Dysexecutive Signs

Dementing illnesses are most notable for the intellectual impairment they cause, such as memory loss, but often they also produce behavioral disturbances such as depression or paranoia. Some also cause physical impairment. Ultimately their severity is best judged by the degree of functional impairment that results from all these factors. Because degenerative dementias such as AD are not yet curable, treatment strategies must be mapped to symptoms. Accurately categorizing the various forms of impairment therefore provides a template for what management strategies to employ. Defining a dementia syndrome therefore must take all these aspects into account.

The mind is like a house with many rooms in it. Memory is one of those rooms, but it is not the whole house. Each room corresponds to a different brain region or set of structures (Fig. 2.1).

This is a useful analogy for patients and for clinicians trying to map a complex and seemingly abstract set of symptoms to a very physically based brain disease. Each room, including the "memory room," is a cognitive domain, and while it is possible to parse the mind many ways, the following four are clinically practical (within the scope of office-based cognitive examination): memory, executive skills, language, and spatial skills. Each domain has "subdomains." Memory includes both verbal (memory for words or verbal material) and spatial (memory for objects or places) memory. Executive skills include working memory (the ability to hold information in the mind's eye, thus permitting multitasking, mental arithmetic, organization of multiple parts, and similar operations), psychomotor speed (the ability to think and act quickly), attention (or the ability to focus on a relevant topic and to shift one's focus when appropriate to avoid perseveration), and judgment. Language includes fluency, comprehension, naming, repetition, reading, and writing. Spatial skills can pertain to any sensory modality but usually are described in relationship to vision (visuospatial perception), construction (constructional praxis), and movement.

Cognitive syndromes that reflect these domains and subdomains, whether in isolation or in combination, include amnesia, aphasia, apraxia, agnosia,

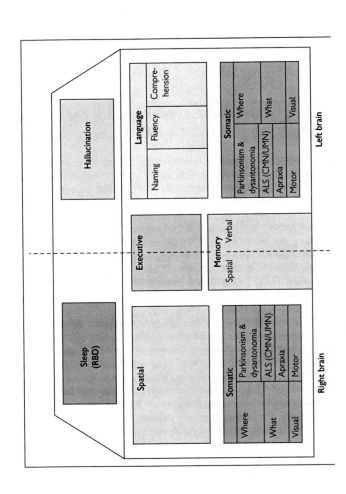

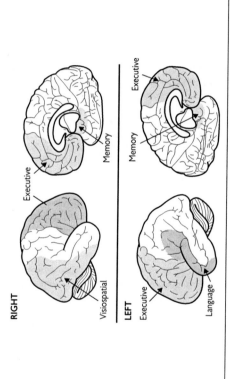

Figure 2.1 Major cognitive domains are like the rooms of a house and correspond to specific brain regions.

psychomotor slowing, and dysexecutive signs. When the severity of impairment becomes disabling, that defines dementia. Amnesia, or memory loss, can be preferentially verbal or spatial in patients with unilateral brain lesions affecting memory-sensitive substrates, but degenerative brain diseases typically affect both due to the usual bilateral involvement of relevant brain structures, including the medial temporal lobe and basal forebrain (the site of central cholinergic nuclei). Aphasia is a language disorder and can be selectively nonfluent (Broca's aphasia), fluent (Wernicke's aphasia), anomic, or mixed (and there are many other subtypes that are less applicable to the dementia setting). Apraxia is a movement disorder, sometimes described as an "aphasia" of learned movement, in which the patient can no longer figure out how to use his or her previously skillful hands to button a shirt, tie shoes, play the piano, draw a picture, and so forth. Although subtypes have been described, the usual form in a dementia setting is called "ideomotor apraxia" due to the inability to translate thought (ideas) into skillful movement. Agnosia is a perceptual disorder, and there are several common manifestations in a dementia setting: anosognosia (the failure to detect and thus deny the existence of one's own illness), prosopagnosia (the failure to recognize familiar faces), and Capgras syndrome (also called reduplicative paramnesia), in which the patient believes familiar people and places to be imposters due to a failure to sense familiarity. Psychomotor slowing, as described above, is a reduction in mental and often physical speed that can manifest as failing to recall a name until later, speaking less, and walking more slowly. This sometimes occurs in the setting of parkinsonism, where the terms "bradyphrenia" and "bradykinesia" have also been used. Dysexecutive syndromes can manifest as excessive distractibility during attentionally demanding tasks (such as digit span and mental arithmetic), poor judgment, obsessive-compulsive and perseverative behaviors (such as pacing and hoarding), or nonstrategic piecemeal approaches to problem solving rather than grasping the larger context.

Defining specifically what domains—that is, which rooms in the house of the mind—are impaired, and to what degree, is one of the major goals of clinical cognitive and neuropsychological assessment. Different dementing diseases produce different patterns of power outages. AD most often begins with an amnestic syndrome, but in a subset of patients it may instead begin as a visual (visual variant AD), aphasic, apraxic, or dysexecutive disorder. Frontotemporal lobar degeneration may cause one of four distinctive disorders: progressive nonfluent aphasia (a language disorder), verbal variant semantic dementia (a severe form of anomia), visual variant semantic dementia (progressive prosopagnosia, the failure to disambiguate familiar faces), and frontotemporal dementia (a dysexecutive syndrome). Vascular dementia often results in mental and physical (psychomotor) slowing, plus dysexecutive symptoms such as poor organization and inability to multitask. Dementia with Lewy bodies also causes psychomotor slowing as well as memory loss and visual disturbances. It is often accompanied by other telltale signs including parkinsonism, visual hallucinations, and REM sleep behavior disorder.

Neuropsychological assessment can help define a cognitive syndrome, but clinicians, especially in the setting of primary care, are the first and sometimes only line of defense against dementia. They need an approach that fits within their time constraints and will still allow them to identify that a potentially disease-related cognitive syndrome exists that requires further diagnosis and treatment. Even when neuropsychological help is available, it is usually easier to determine whether a neuropsychological report confirms a previously suspected diagnosis than to rely on it completely to identify the specific disease. Chapter 3 provides a detailed discussion of cognitive testing, but a few general principles will illustrate how such testing provides the basis for defining patterns of cognitive impairment.

Office-based cognitive testing should follow a standard, methodical approach. Multiple mental status examinations have been published, but by far the most popular is the "Mini-Mental Status Examination" or MMSE (1). One that is used at the Mayo Clinic is the Kokmen (or Short) Test of Mental Status (2). These and others incorporate questions regarding orientation, learning, and memory, a constructional task, some aspect of language, and some form of executive task. They are lacking, however, in tests of psychomotor speed and so can be supplemented with other brief tests, such as the controlled oral word association test (3) or a category fluency task. Both require the patient to recite as many words or objects as possible in a minute. Finally, although many patients with otherwise uncomplicated AD may have no particular physical findings, patients with other forms of dementia may exhibit a tremor or shuffling gait or other feature relevant to the underlying disease process. With such brief measures, it becomes possible to estimate which rooms in the big house of the mind are impaired to what degree, and then to generate an insightful differential diagnosis based upon the ability to match the patient's pattern with known disease-related patterns (Figs. 2.2 and 2.3).

Psychiatric and Related Features

Memory loss may be the most notable feature of AD, but the most disabling aspects of many dementia syndromes are the behavioral problems they cause. Depression and anxiety are diagnostically nonspecific, while visual hallucinations are diagnostically suggestive of dementia with Lewy bodies. Visual hallucinations can also be caused by reversible diseases such as medication toxicity or fungal meningitis, and so their existence should prompt a thorough search for potentially reversible causes. Paranoid delusions, particularly regarding infidelity and theft, commonly occur in patients with AD, although they can also be caused by bipolar disorder and other psychoses. Mania can sometimes manifest in patients with bitemporal degeneration (as occurs in patients with frontotemporal lobar degeneration and AD), but it also may be caused by a toxic-metabolic encephalopathy such as hyponatremia.

Orientation	7/8
Attention	7/7
Learning	4/4
Arithmetic	4/4
Constructions	4/4
Abstractions	3/3
Information	4/4
Recall	0/4
Total	33/38

Letter (or Caretegory) Fluency: unimpaired

Naming: unimpaired

Writing: unimpaired

Simultanagnosia? No

Familiar Faces: unimpaired

History: Memory loss

Physical: unimpaired

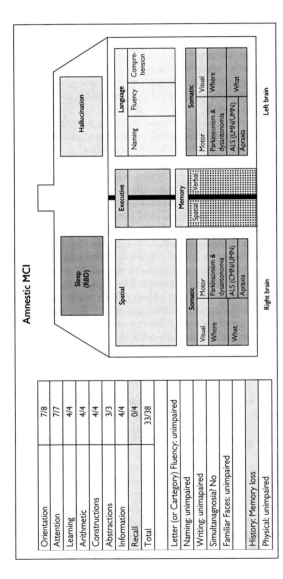

Figure 2.2 Amnestic mild cognitive impairment. Memory is the only cognitive domain impaired on clinical cognitive assessment using the Kokmen Test of Mental Status (2), and this is reflected as only one room in the house of the mind being darkened (that corresponds to the medial temporal lobe, one of the earliest sites for Alzheimer's disease to begin).

Alzheimer's Dementia (Mild)

Orientation	6/8
Attention	7/7
Learning	3/4
Arithmetic	4/4
Constructions	2/4
Abstractions	2/3
Information	3/4
Recall	0/4
Total	27/38

Letter (or Cartegory) Fluency: unimpaired
Naming: mildly impaired
Writing: unimpaired
Simultanagnosia? No
Familiar Faces: unimpaired

History:
  –Memory loss
  –Mild naming difficulty
  –Denies a problem
Physical: unimpaired

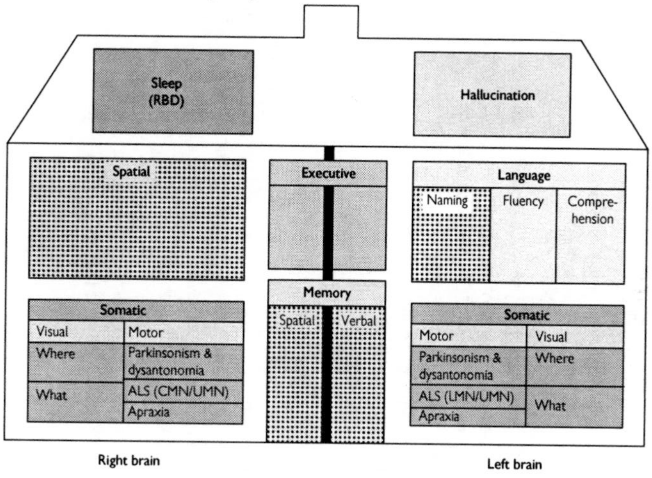

Hallucination

Sleep (RBD)

Spatial

Executive

Memory

Spatial	Verbal

Somatic (Right brain)

Visual	Motor
Where	Parkinsonism & dysantonomia
What	ALS (CMN/UMN)
	Apraxia

Right brain

Language

Naming	Fluency	Compre-hension

Somatic (Left brain)

Motor	Visual
Parkinsonism & dysantonomia	Where
ALS (LMN/UMN)	What
Apraxia	

Left brain

Figure 2.3 Alzheimer's dementia. Multiple cognitive skills are impaired including memory, spatial, and naming resulting in multiple rooms in the house of the mind being darkened that corresponds to more extensive neuropathology.

Less specific but also important is social comportment. Patients with retained social skills are less likely to develop behavioral syndromes, and to casual observers (including unaware physicians) they may appear normal, so that the disability resulting from the underlying intellectual disorder may be severely underestimated. Preservation of social skills and retained insight into one's own level of impairment might seem to be incompatible with the notion of dementia, but insofar as dementia is the disabling impairment of multiple cognitive domains (with or without preservation of the "social skills domain"), there is no inconsistency.

Sleep disorders not only can provide a diagnostic clue as to underlying etiology, but are also a major source of caregiver stress. REM sleep behavior disorder is highly suggestive of a synucleinopathy-based disorder that includes Parkinson's disease (with and without dementia), dementia with Lewy bodies, and multiple system atrophy. Another common sleep disorder is obstructive sleep apnea (OSA). Patients presenting with mild cognitive impairment and prominent daytime fatigue sometimes have OSA rather than a more sinister cause, making OSA a potentially reversible cause of mild memory loss. Other sleep and day–night cycle disturbances such as sundowning are less specific. Sundowning refers to the phenomenon of increased confusion exhibited by many dementia patients as the sun goes down and darkness descends. Also nonspecific are the nocturnal awakenings that may occur either spontaneously or due to another cause such as nocturia. They are an important cause of caregiver stress and so warrant management.

Somatic Signs: Motor and Sensory Disturbances

The prevailing wisdom that dementing illnesses primarily affect the mind and spare the body is an oversimplification. Many physical symptoms and signs are caused by the same degenerative process that produces dementia.

Parkinsonism affects most patients who have dementia with Lewy bodies and, by definition, all patients who have Parkinson's disease with dementia. It is perhaps the most easily identified feature of a "subcortical dementia" whose cognitive profile is defined by prominent psychomotor slowing. Fifty to 75% of patients with dementia in the setting of parkinsonism have AD pathology at autopsy. Less common extrapyramidal diseases that also can result in dementia include progressive supranuclear palsy (impaired vertical eye movements, axial rigidity with prominent backward falls) and Huntington's disease (chorea).

Symptoms and signs of motor neuron disease (amyotrophic lateral sclerosis) include muscle fasciculations, weakness, and frank atrophy and occur in some patients with frontotemporal lobar degeneration (especially the nonfluent aphasia and frontotemporal dementia forms) (4).

Corticobasal ganglionic degeneration is an uncommon but striking disorder that produces severe apraxia and hemirigidity. Though neuropathologically unrelated to AD, it can be mimicked closely enough by AD and by progressive supranuclear palsy to make antemortem diagnosis unreliable. As a rough guide,

Alzheimer apraxic variants tend to have much greater cognitive loss (yet with relatively preserved social skills and insight) and much less rigidity (5).

In addition to motor syndromes, there are also perceptual disorders that characterize certain dementia syndromes. Vision at the level of the cerebral cortex follows two parallel streams: a dorsal parietal stream that maps visual space (the "where" pathway) and a ventral temporal stream important for object recognition (the "what" pathway). Visual variant AD affects the dorsal "where pathway" and causes "simultanagnosia," the inability to map a visual scene in fixed space and time (or a failure to compute visual simultaneity). Despite having normal visual acuity, patients fail to see things in plain sight, especially if the target of interest is embedded in a visually crowded scene. A patient who opens the door of a stuffed refrigerator may fail to see the milk on the shelf right in front of him or her. Patients with corticobasal ganglionic degeneration sometimes have this problem too due to more posterior parietal involvement.

A very different visual syndrome results from degeneration of the ventral "what pathway." Such patients cannot "disambiguate" familiar faces, a syndrome termed prosopagnosia—that is, they can identify a face as a face and its basic characteristics (older man, dark hair, no beard, no glasses) but cannot specify who it is (e.g., President Ronald Reagan). Patients with the visual (right greater than left temporal degeneration) form of semantic dementia, a form of frontotemporal lobar degeneration, manifest this problem. Auditory and tactile disorders also occur but have been less well studied and are usually much more difficult to identify in a clinical setting.

Finally, in the late stage of any degenerative brain disease, physical impairments that commonly arise include dysphagia and gait disturbances that ultimately may cause dehydration, starvation, aspiration, falls, hip fractures (and other injuries), and postoperative complications ultimately leading to death.

Functional Impairment

The definition of disability in patients with dementia is their level of functional impairment, which determines whether they can continue their job, drive, travel, live alone, manage their finances, administer their own medications, cook, feed themselves, dress themselves, bathe themselves, and so forth. While a patient's neurological and cognitive deficits are the primary source of disability, his or her support systems also matter. A patient with a predominantly aphasic disorder may be quite capable of traveling yet cannot speak on the telephone. A patient with visual variant AD may be able to speak on the phone without difficulty but cannot travel. A patient with an amnestic syndrome may have trouble living alone but have no trouble living with a spouse. Finally, the complexity of the environment also matters. A man with mild cognitive impairment who is retired and living in a small town where he is known by all his neighbors can more effectively maintain his premorbid lifestyle than a trial lawyer with a large caseload or an international business traveler.

Each patient's specific pattern of cognitive, behavioral, and physical deficits as well as his or her social setting therefore determines the level of functional impairment. In research settings, tools such as the Clinical Dementia Rating Scale (CDR) (6), the Functional Activities Questionnaire (FAQ), and the Instrumental Activities of Daily Living (IADL) Questionnaire help to quantify functional status, though they are rarely used in clinical practice in part because of the time they consume. Nonetheless, driving, weapons, medication use, living alone, finances, and medical directives must be addressed in early disease stages. Eating, dressing, bathing, and sleeping follow in the middle and later stages, and finally, patient comfort and death with dignity complete the cycle. Many of these issues are managed nonpharmacologically through family and professional caregivers (see Section D).

Timeframe Matters: The Differential Diagnosis of Acute, Subacute, and Chronic Encephalopathy

Diseases evolve over time. Some evolve very quickly, such as a stroke, while others evolve over years, such as AD. When a patient is initially evaluated, however, we are seeing that patient at only one point in time. We rely upon the medical history to define the preceding timeframe and on longitudinal follow-up examinations to ensure that the chronology and semiology of progression fit with our diagnostic expectations. The time course over which a disease evolves has important implications for its potential etiology. Memory loss, for example, may be gradually progressive in onset when caused by AD or abrupt in onset when caused by a tumor.

Dementia is a complex disorder, as our previous discussion of cognitive domains and other categories of dysfunction illustrated. Despite the existence of some characteristic diagnostic patterns, it is easy to mistake any pattern of dementia for another cognitive syndrome. Much is made of the distinction between dementia and delirium, but the two can be very difficult to distinguish from each other. Dementia is characterized by memory loss and delirium by attentional loss, but this is a misleading oversimplification. Memory is often impaired in the setting of delirium, and many patients with dementia have impaired attentional skills. Further, patients with dementia are at heightened risk for delirium, so the two often co-occur.

Rather than attempting to distinguish the two by appearance alone, let us reconsider the timeframe of cognitive impairment. Instead of labeling a patient as demented or delirious, let us use the more general term "encephalopathy." This implies nothing more than a brain disorder, in this case manifesting (though not necessarily exclusively) with impaired cognition. Encephalopathy can be acute/subacute or chronic and can be caused by any pathophysiological category, as illustrated in Table 2.1.

When viewed in this context, AD is a degenerative form of chronic progressive encephalopathy, while a suprasellar craniopharyngioma is a neoplastic form

Table 2.1 Pathophysiological Categories of Acute and Chronic Encephalopathy

	Acute/Subacute	Chronic
Vascular	Stroke	Vascular dementia
Inflammatory	Cerebral vasculitis	Nonvasculitic (NAIM)
Toxic	Alcohol	Prescription medications
Metabolic	Hypoglycemia	Hypothyroidism
Infectious	Herpes encephalitis	Fungal meningitis
Nutritional	Wernicke-Korsakoff	Vitmain B12 deficiency
Degenerative	Creutzfeldt-Jakob disease	Alzheimer's disease
Epileptic	Seizure	Psychomotor status epilepticus
Trauma	Head injury	Dementia pugilisitica
Psychiatric	Psychosis with agitation	Depression
Neoplastic/ Hydrocephalus	Limbic encephalitis	Normal Pressure Hydrocephalus

NAIM, nonvascultic autoimmune inflammatory meningoencephalitis (see Chapter 5)

of acute encephalopathy. Both impair memory and so if viewed together at only one point in time might superficially resemble each other, yet removal of the tumor can restore memory functioning (in at least some patients). In general, the more rapidly progressive a disease, the less likely it is to be degeneratively based, and the more important it becomes to diagnose and treat it before further brain damage and death result.

References

1. Folstein MF, Folstein SE, McHugh PR. Mini-mental state. J Psychiatric Res 1975;12:189–198.

2. Kokmen E, Naessens JM, Offord KP. A short test of mental status: description and preliminary results. Mayo Clin Proc 1987;62:281–288.

3. Benton AL, Hamsher KdeS, Multilingual Aphasia Examination. Iowa City: AJA Associates, 1989.

4. Caselli RJ, Windebank AJ, Petersen RC, et al. Rapidly progressive aphasic dementia and motor neuron disease. Ann Neurol 1993;33(2):200–207.

5. Caselli RJ, Stelmach GE, Caviness JN, et al. A kinematic study of progressive apraxia with and without dementia. Mov Disord 1999;14(2):276–287.

6. Morris JC, Ernesto C, Schafer K, et al. Clinical dementia rating training and reliability in multicenter studies: the Alzheimer's Disease Cooperative Study experience. Neurology 1997;48:1508–1510.

Chapter 3

Diagnostic evaluation of suspected Alzheimer's disease

History and Physical Examination

Confronted by a patient with suspected dementia, there are some key features to identify in the history and on examination. First, AD begins insidiously and progresses gradually. Occasionally, patients or families may report an early "first suspected" event that might give the impression of an abrupt onset. However, continued progression following such events reveals the gradually progressive nature of the disease process.

Second, the most common initial symptom is memory loss, and this remains a prominent deficit throughout the clinical course. Other cognitive deficits are often reported as well. Anomia is a failure to recall the names of familiar people and places, or misnaming a common object. Constructional, spatial, and executive difficulties are reported as difficulties with mechanical household tasks such as operating the television remote control or the microwave oven, or doing a home repair. Anosognosia is the patient's own unawareness or denial of the problem. Sleep disturbances should be sought. Patients with snoring, daytime fatigue, and mild memory difficulties may have sleep apnea, especially if they are also overweight. Falls out of bed and other symptoms of dream enactment behavior should raise suspicion of REM sleep behavior disorder, which commonly accompanies dementia with Lewy bodies and Parkinson's disease. Visual hallucinations also are suspicious for dementia with Lewy bodies (and some forms of reversible encephalopathy).

Third, it is critical to place the patient's symptoms within the context of his or her medical background. Medication use, concurrent systemic illness, prior brain-related diseases, and psychiatric problems can affect the clinical presentation, diagnosis, treatment options, and prognosis. "Dementia" has been cured in a few patients, for example, by stopping their psychoactive and narcotic medications.

Fourth, a family history of dementia in a parent or other relative is common. Though not essential for diagnosis, the absence of a family history in a patient under age 65 years should enhance diagnostic vigilance for other potential causes of cognitive decline. Fifth, pertinent concerns in the social history that either affect or are affected by cognitive impairment include driving habits, whether the patient lives alone or with a potential caregiver, recreational habits (use of tobacco or alcohol, possession of weapons at home), and past educational and occupational history.

Physical and neurological examinations typically reveal no relevant abnormalities in most patients with AD, but a variety of sensorimotor disturbances may appear in Alzheimer variants, in non-Alzheimer forms of dementia, and perhaps most importantly in potentially reversible diseases masquerading as dementia. Among such signs are tremor, gait disturbances, parkinsonism, fasciculations, weakness, muscle atrophy, hemirigidity, apraxia, aphasia, and visual disturbances. Also, because AD usually affects older patients, common comorbidities often need to be weighed for their potential relevance (or lack of relevance). Even if not of direct diagnostic relevance, some comorbid conditions may affect treatment decisions. For example, patients with short bowel syndrome may be at high risk for diarrhea with standard dementia (acetylcholinesterase inhibitor) therapy.

The Mental Status Examination

Mental status testing is the clinician's first step in the objective assessment of the quality and severity of the reported cognitive disturbance. Most types of mental status tests, including the popular Folstein Mini-Mental State Examination (1) and the Kokmen Short Test of Mental Status (2), include questions related to orientation, attention, learning, memory, language, and constructional praxis. Mental status tests ideally should serve three purposes. The first is to generate a global score that will be either above or below a cutoff score that defines it as normal or not. While helpful as a general guide, especially for those who feel uncomfortable with this type of assessment, cutoff scores can be very misleading. Individuals with early-stage disease who are intellectually gifted may "pass" when in fact they have a real problem, while those with low educational backgrounds and poor command of the test language may appear worse than they are. The second and more reliable technique is to establish a baseline level of performance against which future performance may be compared. Whatever confounding factors may exist, they should be equal on each occasion and so subsequent decline may be more accurately determined. Third, mental status testing may provide the more experienced clinician with a pattern of impairment—a sense of which domains are affected and which are spared. This pattern can then be used to determine whether the current profile looks like AD or another disorder.

In addition to "off-the-shelf" mental status tests, it is also useful to have a few other tests available in selected cases. Have the patient write a sentence; to save time, it may be helpful to tell the patient what to write ("Today is a beautiful day"). This allows for the assessment of micrographia as well as aphasic and apraxic agraphia. A timed test, such as letter fluency (asking the patient to recite as many words as possible that begin with the letter S in a minute), or category fluency (name as many animals as possible in a minute), allows for the assessment of mental speed. Age, education, and primary language all influence results. A standard neuropsychology reference can provide such norms for specific tests (such as the Controlled Oral Word Association Test) (3).

Both the Folstein and the Kokmen mental status tests include only verbal memory subtests, so a test of visual memory (such as the Complex Figure Test [3]) is occasionally useful. Visual tests sensitive to the "what" and "where" pathways include famous face recognition (one can use Google Images to generate a group of 5 to 10 photos of recent presidents and movie stars saved on a computer file, or clipped photos from magazines) and a test for simultanagnosia. Simultanagnosia is a disorder in which patients have difficulty seeing specific objects that are surrounded by many others (a defining feature of visual variant AD). An easy way to test for this is to have an old briefcase, drawer, or shoebox with a clutter of common household items such as a soup ladle, an ashtray, a bar of soap, a hairbrush, a comb, and so forth and ask the patient to find the ashtray.

Other aspects of cognitive testing can be improvised, including reading, confrontation naming, aural comprehension, and gestural praxis. For reading, any popular magazine with clear print should suffice, although it is preferable to use stimulus items from actual reading tests (such as the Boston Diagnostic Aphasia Examination [4]). When the patient is reading aloud, listen for paraphasic errors. For naming, use common objects with well-recognized names, such as a button, tie clip, or paperclip. (Do not ask patients to name the parts of a watch, as this is less common than older texts seem to realize and many healthy people do not know what the "stem" is either.) For comprehension, ask patients to show you their left thumb, to touch their left ear with their right thumb, and to show you two fingers on their right hand. Do not simply ask them to squeeze your hands. Not only is this too easy for most aphasic patients, but grasp reflexes can be potentially misinterpreted as a valid response. For gestural praxis, test each arm individually, and use common, easily understood gestures. If a patient runs a hand through her hair when asked to comb her hair, instruct her to pretend she is actually holding a comb and to show how it is used. A toothbrush is another good example. Depending on the time available and level of suspicion, at least five examples of each of these should be completed.

To illustrate a mental status examination more specifically, let us use the Kokmen Test of Mental Status, which is nonproprietary and used at the Mayo Clinic. To administer, it typically takes 5 to 10 minutes in a healthy person, 10 to 15 minutes in amnestic mild cognitive impairment and mild uncomplicated AD, and 20 minutes or so in a patient with psychomotor slowing (dementia with Lewy bodies, Parkinson's disease with dementia, vascular dementia). If this is too long, then a minimal mental status exam (under 5 minutes) should include orientation (date [month, date, year, day of the week, and time] and place [city, state, doctor's office]), learning and remembering three or four words, drawing a clock, and writing a sentence. With the time saved, one could even add a 1-minute test of mental speed (name all the animals). We will explore interpretation of results later.

The following are the eight parts of the Kokmen Test of Mental Status:

1. Orientation: 8 points (month, date, year, day of the week, city, state, building, name)
2. Attention: 7 points (forward digit span up to seven numbers)
3. Learning: 4 points (how many times it takes to repeat four words together; lose one point for each trial after one)
4. Calculation: 4 points (four arithmetic calculations: 14×3, $81 \div 9$, $14 + 17$, $52 - 15$; they may be written)
5. Construction: 4 points (draw a clock and a cube, two points each)
6. Information: 4 points (who was the first president, who is the current president, how many weeks in a year, what is an island)
7. Abstraction: 3 points (what do a cat and dog have in common; what do a blade of grass and a tree have in common; explain "too many cooks spoil the broth")
8. Recall: 4 points (spontaneous, uncued recall of the four words from the learning trial)

The Kokmen Short Test of Mental Status adds up to a maximum score of 38 points, in contrast to the Folstein MMSE, which adds up to 30 points, but the two are similar enough that one can approximate the other.

As described earlier, the mind is like a house with many rooms in it, and different dementias produce different patterns of power outages. Figure 3.1 shows our house to have eight rooms, four of which have two or more subdivisions.

Using these rooms, we can diagnose most of the major dementia syndromes. Each room can be tested with the tools described above that can be done in a physician's office, either by the physician or a trained physician extender. This is not a substitute for more accurate and detailed neuropsychological testing, but it gives the clinician an insightful starting point.

Starting on the first floor, memory is divided into verbal and spatial, corresponding to the left and right cerebral hemispheres. Verbal memory is assessed by learning and recalling four words. Visual memory requires something not included on a mental status test. Convenient tools include the complex figure test (3), or Mesulam's three words/three shapes test (5). In both cases, the patient copies an abstract figure, and after a brief delay is asked to draw it from memory. Flanking the left and right sides of the first floor are the "somatic suites," which contain aspects of vision and movement. Visual functions are assessed on physical examination (visual field testing, looking specifically for an inferior quadrantanopia or visual hemineglect) or with improvised tests for facial recognition (famous faces) and simultanagnosia (the "briefcase test"). Motor functions are all assessed on physical examination, with particular attention to signs of parkinsonism, amyotrophic lateral sclerosis (can include lower motor neuron signs of muscle atrophy, weakness, and fasciculations; upper motor neuron signs of hyperreflexia and spasticity, which is typically asymmetrical; and dysarthria, which is typically mixed with lower motor neuron hypernasality and upper motor neuron strained phonation and slowing of articulation), and apraxia.

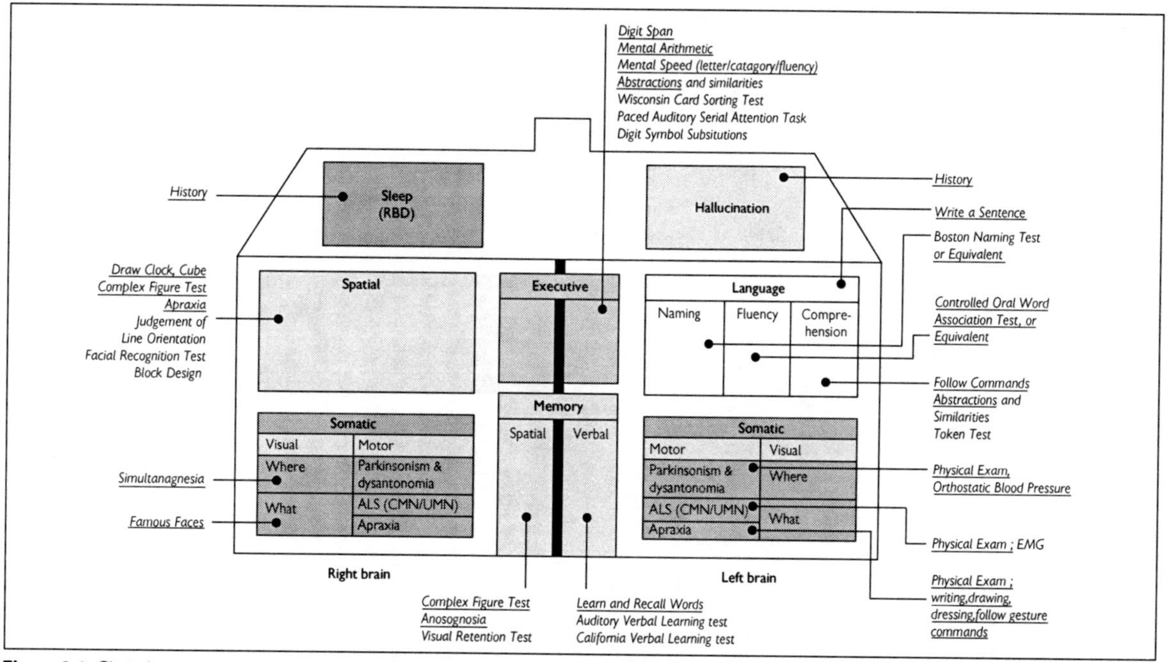

Figure 3.1 Clinical cognitive assessment, including the questions of mental status examinations, probe the different rooms in the house of the mind. Those that are underlined are easily performed in a medical office setting. The others are preferably included in neuropsychological testing.

On the second floor, the spatial room is assessed with clock and cube drawing from the mental status exam, as well as any signs of apraxia. The executive room is assessed with digit span, arithmetic (especially if done mentally), and abstractions from the mental status exam and a timed mental speed test such as letter fluency. The language suite includes naming, fluency, and comprehension. Fluency is readily assessed simply by listening to spontaneous speech. Comprehension requires some specific tasks as described above. Naming is more challenging than it sounds, and again at least five (preferably more) items should be named. Writing a sentence is a language-based task that also is influenced by parkinsonism and apraxia.

On the roof, both sleep (including both obstructive sleep apnea and REM sleep behavior disorder) and hallucinations (typically visual) are assessed by medical history.

While this is not an exhaustive description of the neurological or cognitive examination, it provides an accessible overview with some detailed examples of what is possible in a medical office.

Tests To Consider In All Patients

Brain Imaging

Structural brain imaging with magnetic resonance imaging (MRI) or computed tomography (CT) is essential to assess for relevant structural pathology such as brain tumors, vascular lesions, subdural hematomas, hydrocephalus, and other problems (6). In patients with AD, MRI and CT typically reveal nonspecific, mild to moderate atrophy that may be most pronounced in the most symptomatic regions, especially the medial temporal lobe. Cerebral white matter hyperintensities are a frequent finding in the elderly and are approximately twice as common in patients with dementia than in nondemented elders. While radiologists often refer to these white matter abnormalities as "small vessel ischemic changes" (7), they may also represent secondary degeneration of the white matter from primary cortical neuronal degeneration (8). Quantitative volumetric MRI can track progressive hippocampal atrophy that correlates with symptomatic disease progression (9). Though not usually performed in routine clinical settings, automated algorithms currently under development may provide greater availability of such measurements clinically in the future (10).

Laboratory Assessment

Because there are no widely accepted, highly reliable, commercially available biomarkers for AD, diagnosis rests on clinical recognition of the characteristic syndrome and the assessment of any potentially contributory medical factors (6). The medical factors evaluated should be appropriate for the patient's health history. If a patient is generally healthy, those should still include blood tests for thyroid function, vitamin B12 level, complete blood counts, metabolic function (including tests of liver and renal function, glucose, electrolytes, and calcium). Other tests should be considered as appropriate for the patient's medical background. For example, if a patient has a recent history of lung cancer, then a chest x-ray, erythrocyte sedimentation rate, and contrast-enhanced brain imaging may be appropriate to assess for possibly active metastatic disease. Before cholinesterase inhibitor therapy is prescribed, a baseline electrocardiogram should be obtained to ensure the patient does not have severe conduction abnormalities that might be exacerbated by therapy. These are simply two examples, and not a comprehensive list. Table 2.1 in Chapter 2 lists some of the major pathophysiological categories and gives some examples of diseases in each that present with cognitive impairment.

Patients with unusually rapid symptomatic progression, myoclonus, depressed level of consciousness, or other forms of presentation that would be atypical for AD might be considered for spinal fluid examination. In patients who undergo spinal fluid examination, tests sensitive to infection, malignancy, and inflammatory diseases should be obtained. Electroencephalography can be considered in patients suspected of having seizures, encephalopathic disorders, or rapidly progressive forms of dementia such as Creutzfeldt-Jakob disease. Again, these examples should not be considered exhaustive, and other tests may be appropriate depending upon the specific medical background of a given patient.

Neuropsychological Assessment

To help define the pattern and severity of cognitive loss, neuropsychological testing can supplement the clinical cognitive assessment. The three main questions that neuropsychological assessment can answer are:

1. Is there a problem? This is relevant in patients with mild cognitive impairment (7) and mild dementia, especially when there is disagreement between the patient and others.
2. What is the pattern of difficulty? Different patterns of cognitive impairment correlate with different causes of dementia. This is the "positive" evidence of a specific nosological entity so that the diagnosis of AD is more than just a diagnosis of exclusion.
3. How severe is the problem? Lifestyle changes such as cessation of driving and moving to assisted living are based on the degree of functional impairment, and this in turn correlates with the degree of intellectual impairment disclosed by neuropsychological testing.

Therefore, while useful in almost any patient with dementia, neuropsychological testing can be particularly helpful in assessing mild cases, medicolegally contested cases, and cases where major lifestyle changes will likely be imposed.

Specialized Tests for AD: What Are They and Who Should Get Them?

PET (FDG, PIB) Scans

Structural neuroimaging (CT and MRI) remains the centerpiece of neuroradiological diagnosis because of the critical role it plays in excluding structural lesions and other nondegenerative causes of cognitive decline that can mimic AD. Some investigators have suggested that metabolic imaging with FDG-PET might be of added benefit because it can demonstrate a characteristic pattern of reduced tracer emission in bilateral parietal, temporal, and posterior cingulate regions (11). When the differential diagnosis rests between AD and other degenerative etiologies, particularly frontotemporal dementia, FDG-PET can help to distinguish the two (Fig. 3.2).

In a study that analyzed FDG-PET images from 146 patients with mild to moderate dementia who were subsequently followed for at least 2 years and 139 patients who had postmortem neuropathological assessments an average of 3 years later, FDG-PET readings were associated with about 93% sensitivity and 75% sensitivity in predicting subsequent clinical decline and the neuropathological diagnosis of AD (12). Based on these and other findings, the U.S. Center for Medicare and Medicaid determined that FDG-PET is "reasonable and necessary" in patients with documented cognitive decline and a recently established diagnosis of dementia who meet clinical criteria for both AD and frontotemporal dementia, who have been evaluated for specific alternative neurodegenerative diseases or causative factors, and for whom the cause of the clinical symptoms remains uncertain (Decision Memo CAG-00088R, September 15, 2004).

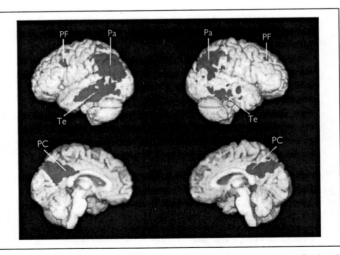

Figure 3.2 Fluorodeoxyglucose positron emission tomography surface map of reduced glucose metabolism in patients with Alzheimer's disease reveals reductions, highlighted, in bilateral parietal, temporal, and posterior cingulate cortices. Reprinted from Eric M. Reiman, M.D., Richard J. Caselli, M.D., Lang S. Yun, et al. Preclinical Evidence of Alzheimer's Disease in Persons Homozygous for the 4 Allele for Apolipoprotein E. NEJM 1996 March; 334(12):752–758. Copyright © [1996] Massachusetts Medical Society. All rights reserved.

Several small studies have suggested that FDG-PET may help predict rates of subsequent cognitive decline and conversion to dementia in patients with mild cognitive impairment, a pathologically heterogeneous group containing many patients with early-stage AD as well as patents with non-Alzheimer etiologies. Most but not all (13) were retrospective in nature and there was some overlap between the PET results of the patients who did and did not subsequently develop dementia. The National Institute on Aging-sponsored Alzheimer's Disease Neuroimaging Initiative is a major, ongoing multicenter study (primarily aimed at MRI and other biomarkers) that includes a PET arm to further evaluate the potential use of FDG-PET in patients with mild cognitive impairment for predicting progression to dementia (14).

More recently, radioligands that bind directly to fibrillar amyloid, a major component of AD neuropathology, have been developed and applied to patients, including Pittsburgh Compound B (PIB; Fig. 3.3) (15,16),

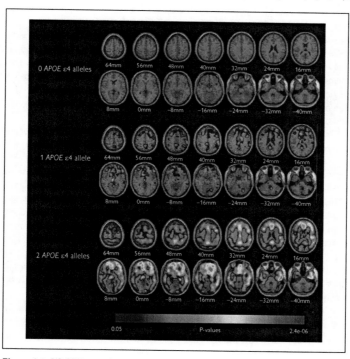

Figure 3.3 PIB-PET scan of asymptomatic 60 year olds with no (top 2 rows), one (middle two rows), and two (bottom two rows) copies of the APOE e4 allele. Colors indicate significance level of fibrillar amyloid deposition which increases in step with e4 gene-dose. This deposition precedes the emergence of clinically symptomatic memory loss by several years. Reprinted from Eric M. Reiman, et al. Fibrillar amyloid-β burden in cognitively normal people at 3 levels of genetic risk for Alzheimer's disease. PNAS 2009; 106:6820–6825.

fluoro-dicyano-dimethylamino-naphthalenyl-propene (FDDNP) (17), and N-methylamino-hydroxystilbene (SB-13) (18), and the SPECT tracer iodo-dim-ethylamino-phenyl-imidazopyridine (IMPY) (18). These represent an important advance in the search for a biomarker of AD so that diagnosis is based on more than exclusionary criteria. However, the extent to which these techniques can be used clinically to predict subsequent clinical decline, to make the histopatho-logical diagnosis of AD, and to guide patient management remains under study.

Cerebrospinal Fluid (CSF) Biomarkers

Also controversial is the use of CSF measurements of β-amyloid (Aβ) and tau proteins as putative biomarkers for AD. Patients with AD have reduced Aβ42 and increased phosphorylated tau in CSF, but there is some overlap between AD and other subject groups (19).

Genetic Testing: Who to Test and Why

Although not yet considered a routine diagnostic procedure for patients with suspected AD, genetic information is increasingly common in medical practice and looms large in the mind of the general public. Relatives of patients frequently ask about the likelihood that AD can be inherited, and about the option of genetic testing of the patient and family members. The genetics of AD are complex, but as with all procedures, the main consideration is the relative risk and benefit of the procedure.

There is a small subset of patients in who genetic testing should be strongly considered. These are patients with early-onset familial AD (EOFAD), which is caused by an autosomal dominant mutation with strong penetrance affect-ing one of three possible genes collectively accounting for less than 5% of all cases of AD. The largest number of mutations are located on the presenilin-1 (PSEN1) gene on chromosome 14, and they are thought to account for the majority of autosomal dominant kindreds (20). A smaller number of mutations have been localized to the amyloid precursor protein (APP) gene on chromo-some 21 (21) and presenilin-2 (PSEN2) on chromosome 1 (22). All result in ele-vated levels of Aβ amyloid, providing powerful evidence for a pathogenetic role of Aβ in the evolution of AD, the "amyloid cascade hypothesis" (23). Typically the age of onset in these cases is under 60 years, and there is usually a strong family history of dementia on one parent's side.

PSEN1 is the only one of these for which there is currently a commercially available genetic test. In suspected EOFAD patients, genetic testing for PSEN1 should be considered to confirm the suspected diagnosis; upon confirmation, PSEN1 testing can be performed in presymptomatic at-risk family members, who may alter important life decisions based on the results. Counseling about possible outcomes, however, should be started before any testing is pursued in order to prepare the patient and especially his or her children for the potential implications of both positive and negative results.

Down syndrome (trisomy 21) is a major cause of mental retardation and has a strong association with AD. If a patient with Down syndrome lives beyond the age of 40 years, there will be neuropathological evidence of AD at autopsy (24). The incidence of progressive dementia increases with age and peaks at roughly 40% to 75% over the age of 60 (24). Analysis of the amyloid plaques has shown that trisomy 21 predisposes to larger plaques, presumably reflecting increased production of Aβ amyloid.

While not an autosomal dominant mutation, the genetic risk factor that accounts for more cases of AD than any other is the APOE e4 allele located on chromosome 19. APOE e4 is associated with late-onset familial and "sporadic" AD, but not autosomal dominant EOFAD (25,26). APOE e4 is a prevalent risk factor for AD, and while the prevalence varies worldwide, it is approximately 20% in North America and Europe (27–29). Each additional copy of the APOE e4 gene reduces the median age of onset of AD but does not appear to strongly influence the rate of cognitive decline in most patients (30–34). APOE e4 homozygotes, however, who represent roughly 2% of the population, may have a slightly faster rate of decline than APOE e4 heterozygotes and noncarriers (35). Several studies have also suggested that APOE genotype may influence the rate of cognitive aging in nondemented individuals (36–40).

In addition to enhancing risk for AD, APOE e4 also correlates with poorer neurological outcome following head trauma (41–43) and intracerebral hemorrhage (44–46). Although it is not known how APOE exerts these effects, possible adverse functional consequences of the e4 isoform compared to the e3 and e2 isoforms include (1) an enhanced rate of cerebral amyloid deposition, (2) reduced protection against oxidative injury, (3) reduced efficiency of synaptic and neuronal repair, (4) reduced neurotrophic properties, possibly related to reduced tau binding causing microtubule destabilization and consequently reduced neurite outgrowth (47), and (5) e4 isoform-specific intraneuronal proteolysis-induced carboxyl fragment toxicity (48–50). These effects are not mutually exclusive and all may be operational to varying degrees.

Deciding whether to perform APOE testing in patients with suspected AD is more problematic. The negative predictive value of APOE e4 is poor, so its absence does not rule out AD. On the other hand, the presence of an APOE e4 allele in a patient with dementia has high positive predictive value for a diagnosis of AD (51). Yet, as discussed, the syndrome of dementia is easily confused with other encephalopathic syndromes, and because APOE e4 is so prevalent, many APOE e4 carriers can develop brain-related illnesses other than AD. Therefore, the presence of an e4 allele does not carry the same diagnostic certainty as a PSEN1 mutation. Regarding management decisions, APOE status does not affect the therapeutic alternatives for a patient with dementia. Therefore, while APOE testing is possible, it is not currently recommended for routine clinical purposes in patients (52). As for asymptomatic relatives, genetic information can be helpful for communication of risk information in the majority of individuals (53), but its use must be questioned given the absence of known effective preventive therapy, and the generally much older age of onset compared to autosomal dominant EOFAD.

In addition to APOE e4, allelic variants of the neuronal sortilin-related receptor (SORL1) gene (54) and the GRB-associated binding protein 2 (GAB2) gene (55), both on chromosome 11, have been associated with late-onset AD. APP, a transmembrane protein, is normally recycled from the cell surface via endocytosis. When SORL1 is underexpressed, APP is sorted into Aβ-generating endocytic compartments (54). GAB2 is a scaffolding protein that interacts with APOE e4 to further modify risk (55). The search for additional susceptibility genes for late-onset AD continues, and some studies have raised the possibility of additional genetic loci on chromosomes 10 (56) and 12 (57). Also, weaker genetic risk factors in cholesterol and glucose metabolic pathways may further influence the cumulative genetic risk for late-onset and sporadic AD (58–61). Currently there are no commercially available tests for any of these genes. The recently developed AlzGene database aims to provide a publicly available and regularly updated review of AD genetic linkage and association studies (http://www.alzforum.org/res/com/gen/alzgene/).

Concluding It's AD: Summary

The diagnosis of AD depends on the positive evidence of a clinical syndrome that looks like AD: gradually progressive memory loss over the course of many months to several years with the gradual emergence of aphasia, agnosia, and apraxia with or without additional behavioral features, including sundowning and paranoia. The bulk of the diagnostic evaluation is made up of tests that provide "negative" support, specifically structural brain imaging (CT or MRI), and blood tests for commonly encountered potentially reversible diseases, including thyroid function tests and vitamin B12 levels. Additionally, complete blood counts and a basic metabolic panel (including serum electrolytes, calcium, blood urea nitrogen, creatinine, glucose, and liver chemistries) should be checked. In mild cases posing diagnostic uncertainty, when lifestyle changes are likely to be needed, when medicolegal issues may arise, or under other circumstances, neuropsychological testing can also be useful. Some Alzheimer-specific tests can provide additional positive support for the diagnosis, including FDG-PET, CSF levels of amyloid and tau proteins, and genetic tests (such as APOE), but they are costly, their benefit remains in doubt, and they are not currently recommended for routine clinical diagnosis and management.

Ultimately, when a diagnosis of AD is made, it should be understood by the family and provider that the disease is not curable at present, is invariably progressive, and in the absence of other supervening illness is ultimately fatal, thus warranting this diagnostic rigor.

References

1. Folstein MF, Folstein SE, McHugh PR. Mini-mental state. J Psychiatric Res 1975;12:189–198.

2. Kokmen E, Naessens JM, Offord KP. A short test of mental status: description and preliminary results. Mayo Clin Proc 1987;62:281–288.

3. Lezak MD, Howieson DB, Loring DW. Neuropsychological Assessment, 4th ed. New York: Oxford University Press, 2004.

4. Goodglass H, Kaplan E. Boston Naming Test. Philadelphia: Lippincott Williams & Wilkins, 2000.

5. Mesulam MM. Principles of Behavioral and Cognitive Neurology, 2nd ed. New York: Oxford University Press, 2000.

6. Knopman DS, DeKosky ST, Cummings JL, et al. Practice parameter: diagnosis of dementia (an evidence-based review): report of the Quality Standards Subcommittee of the American Academy of Neurology. Neurology 2001;56:1143–1153.

7. Young VG, Halliday GM, Kril JJ. Neuropathologic correlates of white matter hyperintensities. Neurology 2008;71:804–811.

8. Matsusue E, Sugihara S, Fujii S, et al. Wallerian degeneration of the corticospinal tracts: postmortem MR-pathologic correlations. Acta Radiol 2007;48:690–694.

9. Jack CR Jr, Shiung MM, Weigand DS, et al. Brain atrophy rates predict subsequent clinical conversion in normal elderly and amnestic MCI. Neurology 2005;65:1227–1231.

10. Morra JH, Tu Z, Apostolova LG, et al. Automated 3D mapping of hippocampal atrophy and its clinical correlates in 400 subjects with Alzheimer's disease, mild cognitive impairment, and elderly controls. Hum Brain Mapp 2009; Jan 26 (Epub).

11. Mosconi L, Tsui WH, Herholz K, et al. Multicenter standardized 18F-FDG PET diagnosis of mild cognitive impairment, Alzheimer's disease, and other dementias. J Nucl Med 2008;49:390–398.

12. Hoffman JM, Welsh-Bohmer KA, Hanson M, et al. FDG PET imaging in patients with pathologically verified dementia. J Nucl Med 2000;41:1920–1928.

13. Drzezga A, Grimmer T, Riemenschneider M, et al. Prediction of individual clinical outcome in MCI by means of genetic assessment and (18)F-FDG PET. J Nucl Med 2005;46:1625–1632.

14. Mueller SG, Weiner MW, Thal LJ, et al. The Alzheimer's Disease Neuroimaging Initiative. Neuroimaging Clin North Am 2005;15:869.

15. Klunk WE, Engler H, Nordberg A, et al. Imaging brain amyloid in Alzheimer's disease with Pittsburgh Compound B. Ann Neurol 2004;55:306–319.

16. Mathis CA, Wang Y, Holt DP, et al. Synthesis and evaluation of 11C-labeled 6-substituted 2-arylbenzothiazoles as amyloid imaging agents. J Med Chem 2003;46:2740–2754.

17. Shoghi-Jadid K, Small GW, Agdeppa ED, et al. Localization of neurofibrillary tangles and beta-amyloid plaques in the brains of living patients with Alzheimer disease. Am J Geriatr Psychiatry 2002;10:24–35.

18. Kung MP, Hou C, Zhuang ZP, et al. Binding of two potential imaging agents targeting amyloid plaques in postmortem brain tissues of patients with Alzheimer's disease. Brain Res 2004;1025:98–105.

19. Sunderland T, Linker G, Mirza N, et al. Decreased beta-amyloid1–42 and increased tau levels in cerebrospinal fluid of patients with Alzheimer disease. JAMA 2003;289:2094–2103.

20. Sherrington R, Rogaev EI, Liang Y, et al. Cloning of a gene bearing missense mutations in early-onset familial Alzheimer's disease. Nature 1995;375:754–760.

21. Goate A, Chartier-Harlin MC, Mullan M, et al. Segregation of a missense mutation in the amyloid precursor protein gene with familial Alzheimer's disease. Nature 1991;349:704–706.

22. Levy-Lahad E, Wasco W, Poorkaj P, et al. Candidate gene for the chromosome 1 familial Alzheimer's disease locus. Science 1995;269:973–977.

23. Hardy JA, Higgins GA. Alzheimer's disease: the amyloid cascade hypothesis. Science 1992;256:184–185.

24. Wisniewski KE, Wisniewski HM, Wen GY. Occurrence of neuropathological changes and dementia of Alzheimer's disease in Down's syndrome. Ann Neurol 1985;17:278–282.

25. Corder EH, Saunders AM, Strittmatter WJ, et al. Gene dose of apolipoprotein E type 4 allele and the risk of Alzheimer's disease in late onset families. Science 1993;261:921–923.

26. Saunders AM, Strittmatter WJ, Schmechel D, et al. Association of apolipoprotein E allele epsilon 4 with late-onset familial and sporadic Alzheimer's disease. Neurology 1993;43:1467–1472.

27. Gerdes LU, Klausen IC, Sihm I, et al. Apolipoprotein E polymorphism in a Danish population compared to findings in 45 other study populations around the world. Genet Epidemiol 1992;9:155–167.

28. Corbo RM, Scacchi R. Apolipoprotein E (APOE) allele distribution in the world: is APOE*4 a "thrifty" allele? Ann Hum Genet 1999;63:301–310.

29. Zekraoui L, Lagarde JP, Raisonnier A, et al. High frequency of the apolipoprotein E *4 allele in African pygmies and most of the African populations in sub-Saharan Africa. Hum Biol 1997;69:575–581.

30. Basun H, Grut M, Winblad B, et al. Apolipoprotein epsilon 4 allele and disease progression in patients with late-onset Alzheimer's disease. Neurosci Lett 1995;183:32–34.

31. Dal FG, Rasmusson DX, Brandt J, et al. Apolipoprotein E genotype and rate of decline in probable Alzheimer's disease. Arch Neurol 1996;53:345–350.

32. Gomez-Isla T, West HL, Rebeck GW, et al. Clinical and pathological correlates of apolipoprotein E epsilon 4 in Alzheimer's disease. Ann Neurol 1996;39:62–70.

33. Kurz A, Egensperger R, Haupt M, et al. Apolipoprotein E epsilon 4 allele, cognitive decline, and deterioration of everyday performance in Alzheimer's disease. Neurology 1996;47:440–443.

34. Growdon JH, Locascio JJ, Corkin S, et al. Apolipoprotein E genotype does not influence rates of cognitive decline in Alzheimer's disease. Neurology 1996;47:444–448.

35. Craft S, Teri L, Edland SD, et al. Accelerated decline in apolipoprotein E-epsilon4 homozygotes with Alzheimer's disease. Neurology 1998;51:149–153.

36. Jonker C, Schmand B, Lindeboom J, et al. Association between apolipoprotein E epsilon4 and the rate of cognitive decline in community-dwelling elderly individuals with and without dementia. Arch Neurol 1998;55:1065–1069.

37. Caselli RJ, Graff-Radford NR, Reiman EM, et al. Preclinical memory decline in cognitively normal apolipoprotein E-epsilon4 homozygotes. Neurology 1999;53:201–207.

38. Caselli RJ, Osborne D, Reiman EM, et al. Preclinical cognitive decline in late middle-aged asymptomatic apolipoprotein E-e4/4 homozygotes: a replication study. J Neurol Sci 2001;189:93–98.

39. Baxter LC, Caselli RJ, Johnson SC, et al. Apolipoprotein E epsilon 4 affects new learning in cognitively normal individuals at risk for Alzheimer's disease. Neurobiol Aging 2003;24:947–952.

40. Caselli RJ, Reiman EM, Osborne D, et al. Longitudinal changes in cognition and behavior in asymptomatic carriers of the APOE e4 allele. Neurology 2004;62:1990–1995.

41. Sorbi S, Nacmias B, Piacentini S, et al. ApoE as a prognostic factor for posttraumatic coma. Nat Med 1995;1:852.

42. Jordan BD, Relkin NR, Ravdin LD, et al. Apolipoprotein E epsilon4 associated with chronic traumatic brain injury in boxing. JAMA 1997;278:136–140.

43. Friedman G, Froom P, Sazbon L, et al. Apolipoprotein E-epsilon4 genotype predicts a poor outcome in survivors of traumatic brain injury. Neurology 1999;52:244–248.

44. Alberts MJ, Graffagnino C, McClenny C, et al. ApoE genotype and survival from intracerebral haemorrhage. Lancet 1995;346:575.

45. MCarron MO, Muir KW, Weir CJ, et al. The apolipoprotein E epsilon4 allele and outcome in cerebrovascular disease. Stroke 1998;29:1882–1887.

46. McCarron MO, Hoffmann KL, DeLong DM, et al. Intracerebral hemorrhage outcome: apolipoprotein E genotype, hematoma, and edema volumes. Neurology 1999;53:2176–2179.

47. Horsburgh K, McCarron MO, White F, et al. The role of apolipoprotein E in Alzheimer's disease, acute brain injury and cerebrovascular disease: evidence of common mechanisms and utility of animal models. Neurobiol Aging 2000;21:245–255.

48. Harris FM, Brecht WJ, Xu Q, et al. Carboxyl-terminal-truncated apolipoprotein E4 causes Alzheimer's disease-like neurodegeneration and behavioral deficits in transgenic mice. Proc Natl Acad Sci USA 2003;100:10966–10971.

49 Brecht WJ, Harris FM, Chang S, et al. Neuron-specific apolipoprotein e4 proteolysis is associated with increased tau phosphorylation in brains of transgenic mice. J Neurosci 2004;24:2527–2534.

50. Huang Y, Weisgraber KH, Mucke L, et al. Apolipoprotein E: diversity of cellular origins, structural and biophysical properties, and effects in Alzheimer's disease. J Mol Neurosci 2004;23:189–204.

51. Nalbantoglu J, Gilfix BM, Bertrand P, et al. Predictive value of apolipoprotein E genotyping in Alzheimer's disease: results of an autopsy series and an analysis of several combined studies. Ann Neurol 1994;36:889–895.

52. Knopman DS, DeKosky ST, Cummings JL, et al. Practice parameter: diagnosis of dementia (an evidence-based review): report of the Quality Standards Subcommittee of the American Academy of Neurology. Neurology 2001;56:1143–1153.

53. Roberts JS, Cupples LA, Relkin NR, et al. Genetic risk assessment for adult children of people with Alzheimer's disease: the Risk Evaluation and Education for Alzheimer's Disease Study (REVEAL). J Ger Psychiatry Neurol 2005;18:250–255.

54. Rogaeva E, Meng Y, Lee JH, et al. The neuronal sortilin-related receptor SORL1 is genetically associated with Alzheimer disease. Nat Genet 2007;39:168–177.

55. Reiman EM, Webster JA, Myers AJ, et al. GAB2 alleles modify Alzheimer's risk in APOE epsilon4 carriers. Neuron 2007;54(5):713–720.

56. Hamshere ML, Holmans PA, Avramopoulos D, et al. Genome-wide linkage analysis of 723 affected relative pairs with late-onset Alzheimer's disease. Hum Mol Genet 2007;16:2703–2712.

57. Beecham GW, Martin ER, Li YJ, et al. Genome-wide association study implicates a chromosome 12 risk locus for late-onset Alzheimer disease. Am J Hum Genet 2009;84:35–43.

58. Papassotiropoulos A, Streffer JR, Tsolaki M, et al. Increased brain beta-amyloid load, phosphorylated tau, and risk of Alzheimer disease associated with an intronic CYP46 polymorphism. Arch Neurol 2003;60:29–35.

59. Johansson A, Katzov H, Zetterberg H, et al. Variants of CYP46A1 may interact with age and APOE to influence CSF Abeta42 levels in Alzheimer's disease. Hum Genet 2004;114:581–587.

60. Wang B, Zhang C, Zheng W, et al. Association between a T/C polymorphism in intron 2 of cholesterol 24S-hydroxylase gene and Alzheimer's disease in Chinese. Neurosci Lett 2004;369:104–107.

61. Papassotiropoulos A, Fountoulakis M, Dunckley T, et al. Genetics, transcriptomics, and proteomics of Alzheimer's disease. J Clin Psychiatry 2006;67:652–670.

Chapter 4

When it's not Alzheimer's disease: four brief illustrative cases of reversible "dementias"

The following four examples are an attempt to bring to life what may all too often seem a more theoretical than real possibility of a reversible dementia. There are many more causes of reversible dementia than the diseases represented by these four cases, but the principles of diagnosis are similar. Because the frequency of reversible dementia depends entirely on its definition, it is difficult to accurately judge frequency, but an overall estimate might place it at roughly 10% to 15% of patients presenting with what might appear initially to be a dementia syndrome (1). Cognitive side effects of medications are very common and should always be considered. Similarly, hypothyroidism and vitamin B12 deficiency are very common, so these must be considered in any patient with cognitive complaints, although in our experience they are less often a cause of dementia than the less common diseases illustrated in this chapter.

Drug-Induced Chronic Encephalopathy

A 72-year-old retired businessman with a history of bipolar disorder presented with a 2-year history of mild gait decline and a 7-month history of memory decline. His father died of amyotrophic lateral sclerosis. His sister had bipolar disorder and his brother had Parkinson's disease. Medications included a stable dose of lithium with an elevated blood level of 1.6 (therapeutic range 0.9–1.2 mg/dL). On examination, he had prominent memory difficulties and scored 18/30 on the MMSE. He had pronounced cognitive slowing, producing only seven words in 3 minutes on a timed letter fluency test. Posture was stooped. He had a mildly shuffling gait and rest tremor consistent with parkinsonism. Modest reduction of his lithium dose as well as trials of donepezil and levodopa produced little benefit. He was hospitalized and all medications, including lithium, were discontinued. Over the following 3 days his cognitive status returned to normal, including memory and psychomotor speed. On repeat examination his MMSE was 29/30 and he produced 30 words on the same timed letter fluency test over 3 minutes (Fig. 4.1).

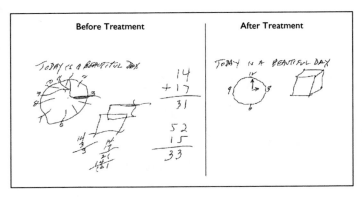

Figure 4.1 Clock and cube constructions before and after discontinuation of Lithium in a 72 year old man with a chronic toxic encephalopathy masqerading as dementia.

His parkinsonism also improved, but over the next several years it continued to modestly worsen despite his ongoing normal cognitive state.

The combination of a subcortical pattern of dementia (manifested by psychomotor slowing) and parkinsonism is suggestive of a synucleinopathy such as dementia with Lewy bodies or Parkinson's disease with dementia, and the additional family history not only reinforces this notion but also adds the possibility of an inheritable disorder such as a tau gene mutation (2). Lithium may induce a toxic encephalopathy, especially in combination with a neuroleptic agent (3–5), and in our patient, progressive dopaminergic deficiency due to recent-onset Parkinson's disease may have been a precipitating factor. Any psychoactive medication should be considered suspect in the setting of impaired cognition.

Fungal Meningitis

A 66-year-old insulin-dependent diabetic, hypertensive man with mild memory concerns underwent induction of general anesthesia for a planned laparoscopic cholecystectomy but developed bradycardia (into the 30s) and hypotension requiring fluid and pressor resuscitation over 10 minutes. The surgery was cancelled, and he was discharged home 2 days later. Over the next two months his thinking became "foggier" and he developed a slow, shuffling gait. On examination he had significant mental slowing on a letter fluency test and had severe memory loss. He had stooped posture and a shuffling gait, but no tremor. An MRI of the brain showed ventricular enlargement suggestive of normal-pressure hydrocephalus, and he underwent serial spinal taps with videotaped and timed gait before and after to assess his response to CSF withdrawal. Although his gait failed to improve with CSF removal, the CSF itself was abnormal, and

Table 4.1 Neuropsychology

	2-27-04	4-6-05	6-14-06
VC	98	98	96
PO*	97	101	105
WMI*	106	109	115
PSI	86	91	84
AVLT-TL	32	31	33
AVLT-LTM	0	1	2
BNT*	47	53	54
COWA*	19	18	30
TOKEN*	35	42	43
TMT-A (s)*	45	31	37
TMT-B (s)*	210	85	99

VC, Verbal Comprehension; PO, Perceptual Organization; WMI, Working Memory Index; PSI, Processing Speed Index (VC, PO, WMI, and PSI are all derived from the Wechsler Adult Intelligence Scale-III); AVLT, Auditory Verbal Learning Test; TL, Total Learning; LTM, Long-Term Memory; BNT, Boston Naming Test; COWA, Controlled Oral Word Association Test; TOKEN, Token Test; TMT, Trail Making Test (Parts A and B); s, seconds. Tests marked with an asterisk improved with treatment.

Table 4.2 CSF

	3-19-04	6-16-04	10-18-04	4-4-05	5-25-06
Protein	189	143	136	113	111
Glucose	64/154	73/252	104/142	72/160	53/65
WBC	134	97	64	12	–
OB	10	–	–	12	5
IgGindex	1.8	1.84	1.43	1.24	0.93
IgG syn r	192.5	129.9	92.2	68.3	36.7
Cocci titre	1:16	1:8	1:4	1:4	–

OB, oligoclonal bands; IgG syn r, IgG synthesis rate.

a diagnosis of fungal meningitis due to *Coccidioides immitis* ("Valley fever") was made. He was treated with the antifungal agent fluconazole 400 mg bid, and both cognition and gait gradually improved back to baseline.

The most common causes of fungal meningitis are Cryptococcus, *Histoplasma capsulatum*, and *C. immitis* (6). Coccidioidomycosis, or San Joaquin Valley fever, is endemic to the American Southwest. It usually causes a self-limited respiratory infection reported in 100,000 cases annually, but approximately 60% of those infected are asymptomatic. Arizona reported an increase of 54% over a 4-year period between 1998 and 2001 (7). An extrapulmonary disseminated form can involve skin, lymph nodes, bones, joints, and the central nervous system. Under 100 cases of cocci meningitis are reported each year, but without treatment, 90% of the patients may die within a year (8). Symptoms include headache (in 75%) and rapidly progressing cognitive decline, but it can also present insidiously, mimicking normal-pressure hydrocephalus (9). Lifelong treatment with oral fluconazole is recommended because of the high rate of relapse (10,11). With treatment, clinical signs of response may take several weeks, and CSF improvement typically lags symptomatic improvement. (This case has been published previously [12].)

Autoimmune Encephalopathy

A 56-year-old woman developed progressive personality changes and confusion that fluctuated in severity over 7 months. She began chain-smoking cigarettes, drinking voluminous amounts of wine, and walking in the snow barefoot, and on one occasion she attempted to exit a moving car. On examination she scored 21/30 on the MMSE. She had a mild static tremor and unsteady gait with normal steppage and base. Laboratory studies revealed an elevated antineutrophil cytoplasmic antibody and a mild CSF lymphocytic pleocytosis (11 WBC), with mildly elevated total protein and IgG synthesis levels. A right prefrontal leptomeningeal and brain biopsy revealed low-grade perivascular lymphocytic inflammatory infiltrates (Fig. 4.2).

A course of oral corticosteroid therapy resulted in modest but only transient improvement lasting several days. With the addition of cyclophosphamide, restoration of normal baseline personality and cognitive functioning was achieved over nearly a year (Fig. 4.3 and Table 4.3). Three years later she remains well off all medications and free of dementia.

This patient had a nonvasculitic autoimmune inflammatory meningoencephalopathy (NAIM). Several autoimmune-mediated meningoencephalitides have been described under diverse names and presumed etiologies. This was originally labeled as Hashimoto's encephalopathy, reflecting the original association with thyroid autoimmunity (13), but multiple serological associations have since been described (14). Presentation can be acute, subacute, or chronic. Response to steroids is generally (but as this case illustrates not invariably) robust (15). In addition to serological evidence of autoimmunity, CSF abnormalities will usually support the clinical suspicion. While an exceptional patient may have meningeal enhancement, there are no diagnostically reliable radiological signs. Electroencephalography (EEG) can show severe but nonspecific slowing, but this too is not invariable. When suspected, serological evidence of an autoimmune state, EEG evidence of encephalopathy, and CSF evidence of intrathecal inflammation, including IgG index and synthesis rate, should be sought. A brief (2 week) course of empirical corticosteroid therapy can be a reasonable diagnostic step in many patients, but unless the response is robust, ultimately the diagnosis may require a brain biopsy. Treatment should begin with high-dose corticosteroids, and a rapid (days), clinically evident response should be anticipated, but in patients with histopathological confirmation in whom steroid

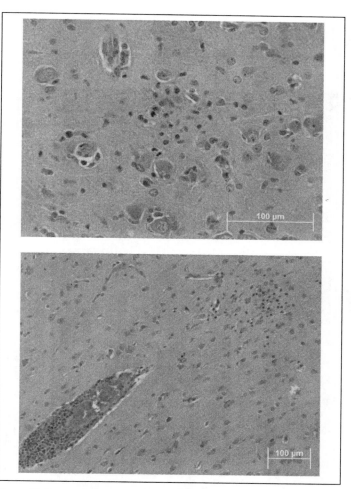

Figure 4.2 Nonvasculitic autoimmune inflammatory meningoencephalitis causing a steroid-responsive chronic progressive encephalopathy masquerading as rapidly progressive dementia in a 56 year old woman. Note increased numbers of cytologically normal lymphocytes in brain parenchyma and surrounding a blood vessel. There no frank vessel wall invasion or necrosis, and so this is not vasculitis. Reprinted from Lyons MK, Caselli RJ, Parisi JE. Nonvasculitic autoimmune inflammatory meningoencephalitis as a cause of potentially reversible dementia: report of 4 cases. J Neurosurg 2008 May; 108(5):1024–7.

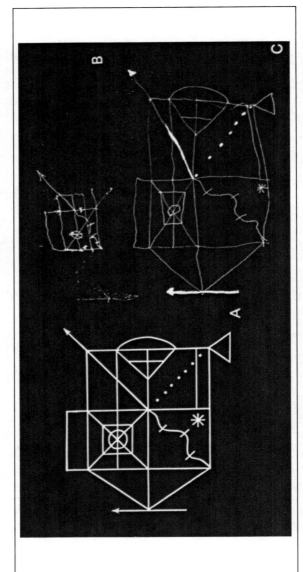

Figure 4.3 Taylor Complex Figure (A). The patient's attempted copy of this design at the time of her presentation (B) is severly impaired, but after only a month of steroid treatment has improved to normal (C), though it would continue to improve even more in subsequent months. Caselli RJ, Scheithauer BW, O'Duffy JD, Peterson GC, Westmoreland BF, Davenport PA. Chronic inflammatory meningoencephalitis should not be mistaken for Alzheimer's disease. Mayo Clin Proc 1993 Sep;68:846–853.

KTMS	Baseline	2 months	19 months
Orientation	7/8	8/8	8/8
Attention	4/7	6/7	7/7
Learning	4/4	4/4	4/4
Calculation	0/4	2/4	4/4
Information	4/4	4/4	4/4
Abstraction	2/3	3/3	3/3
Construction	2/4	1//4	4/4
Recall	3//4	3//4	4/4
Total	26/38	30/38	38/38

Table 4.3 Serial mental status performance with therapy

therapy is insufficient, addition of cyclophosphamide or another cytotoxic agent (as would be used for cerebral vasculitis treatment [15]) should be considered. Erythrocyte sedimentation rate, EEG, and clinical cognitive assessment are helpful to monitor a patient's therapeutic course.

Craniopharyngioma

A 55-year-old woman with a history of escalating headaches over several months began to note memory loss that interfered with her daily activities. Her husband also noted a personality change, with greater apathy, complacency, and emotional indifference. On examination, she had memory difficulties (MMSE was 27/30 with 0/3 on delayed recall) with relative preservation of other cognitive domains. Her MRI showed an enhancing mass in the suprasellar region compatible with a craniopharyngioma, and she underwent surgical removal (Fig. 4.4). Postoperatively, her memory returned to normal, but her personality changes persisted.

Suprasellar masses compress several salient memory substrates, including the fornices (one of two major efferent pathways of the hippocampal formation), their septal and hypothalamic targets, and the cholinergic basal forebrain nuclei. Amnestic syndromes caused by craniopharyngiomas have been described (16) but are uncommon. At least one study was able to demonstrate disruption of both the postcommissural fornix and the mammillothalamic tract as the probable basis for this (17). Our experience and isolated case reports suggest that the amnestic syndrome is potentially reversible. Not all patients described have made a complete recovery (18), however, and some have suffered memory loss as a consequence of the surgery itself (19).

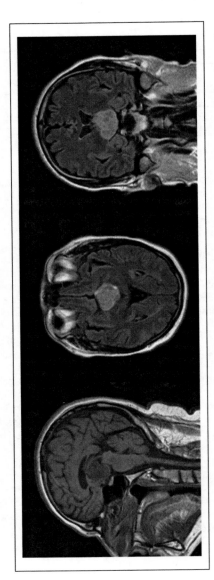

Figure 4.4 Craniopharyngioma in suprasellar region compressing hypothalamus and local structures producing amnestic syndrome and personality changes.

References

1. Katzman R. Diagnosis and management of dementia. In Katzman R, Rowe JW, eds. Principles of Geriatric Neurology. Philadelphia: FA Davis, 1992:167–206.

2. Lynch T, Sano M, Marder KS, et al. Clinical characteristics of a family with chromosome 17-linked disinhibition-dementia-parkinsonism-amyotrophy complex. Neurology 1994;44:1878–1884.

3. Boora K, Xu J, Hyatt J. Encephalopathy with combined lithium-risperidone administration. Acta Psychiatr Scand 2008;117:394–395.

4. Kaplan PW, Birbeck G. Lithium-induced confusional states: nonconvulsive status epilepticus or triphasic encephalopathy? Epilepsia 2006;47:2071–2074.

5. Fetzer J, Kader G, Danahy S. Lithium encephalopathy: a clinical, psychiatric, and EEG evaluation. Am J Psychiatry 1981;138:1622–1623.

6. Roos KL. Brain infections. In Rizzom E, Eslinger PJ, eds. Principles and Practices of Behavioral Neurology and Neuropsychology. Philadelphia: WB Saunders, 2004:513–515.

7. Centers for Disease Control and Prevention. Increase in coccidioidomycosis—Arizona, 1998–2001. Morbidity and Mortality Weekly Report 2003;52(6):109–112.

8. Stevens DA. Current concepts: coccidioidomycosis. N Engl J Med 1995;332(16):1077–1082.

9. Crum NF, Lederman ER, Stafford CM, et al. Coccidioidomycosis: a descriptive survey of a reemerging disease. Clinical characteristics and current controversies. Medicine 2004;83(3):149–175.

10. Dewsnup DH, Galgiani JN, Graybill JR, et al. Is it ever safe to stop azole therapy for Coccidioides immitis meningitis? Ann Intern Med 1996;124:305.

11. Deresinski SC. Coccidioidomycosis; efficacy of new agents and future prospects. Curr Op Infect Dis 2001;14(6):693–696.

12. Hoffman Snyder C. Coccidioidal meningitis presenting as memory loss. J Am Acad Nurse Pract 2005;17:181–186.

13. Brain L, Jellinek EH, Ball K. Hashimoto's disease and encephalopathy. Lancet 1966;2:512–514.

14. Caselli RJ, Boeve BF, Scheithauer BW, et al. Nonvasculitic autoimmune inflammatory meningoencephalitis (NAIM): a reversible form of encephalopathy. Neurology 1999;53(7):1579–1581.

15. Caselli RJ, Hunder GG. Temporal arteritis and cerebral vasculitis. In Johnson RT, Griffin JW, eds. Current Therapy in Neurologic Disease 4. St. Louis: Mosby-Year Book, 1993:196–201.

16. Kupers RC, Fortin A, Astrup J, et al. Recovery of anterograde amnesia in case of craniopharyngioma. Arch Neurol 2004;61:1948–1952.

17. Saeki N, Sunami K, Kubota M, et al. Heavily T2-weighted MR imaging of white matter tracts in the hypothalamus: normal and pathologic demonstrations. Am J Neuroradiol 2001;22:1468–1475.

18. Tanaka Y, Miyazawa Y, Akaoka F, Yamada T. Amnesia following damage to the mammillary bodies. Neurology 1997;48:160–165.

19. Chakrabarti I, Amar AP, Couldwell W, et al. Long-term neurological, visual, and endocrine outcomes following transnasal resection of craniopharyngioma. J Neurosurg 2005;102:650–657.

Alzheimer's disease and its clinical syndromes

A given disease may express itself in a variety of ways. Tuberculosis, for example, most often causes pneumonia, but it can also cause osteomyelitis. A patient with a cerebral infarction in Broca's area presents a very different syndrome than one whose infarction involves the right parietal lobe. This principle has been generally understood for most disease categories, but less so for degenerative diseases. However, neurodegenerative diseases in general, and AD in particular, also follow this principle. There are a variety of clinical syndromes that may result from AD, and while this might seem confusing, we can start by realizing that the terms Alzheimer's disease and Alzheimer's dementia are not synonymous. Alzheimer's disease is a specific disease process with a characteristic and defining neuropathological signature. The syndromes this disease produces, however, vary. The best-recognized and most commonly manifested clinical syndrome produced by AD is Alzheimer's dementia, and it is characterized by severe memory loss with milder degrees of aphasia, apraxia, agnosia, and certain personality changes. But AD may also cause predominantly aphasic, apraxic, agnostic, or dysexecutive patterns of dementia bearing little resemblance to the more typical syndrome.

AD, as a neuropathologically defined entity, can also co-occur with other common age-related neuropathologies, including Parkinson's disease, cerebral infarction, and amyloid angiopathy. Therefore, the notion of AD as a pathologically and clinically well-demarcated entity is a misleading oversimplification. To understand AD, we must become familiar with its range of clinical manifestations and the neuropathological company it keeps.

Chapter 5

The neurobiology of Alzheimer's disease

Neuropathology

AD is a degenerative brain disease whose defining microscopic features are the amyloid plaque and the neurofibrillary tangle. Amyloid plaque formation is generally thought to precede (1) and ultimately cause neurofibrillary tangle formation. Cognitive decline parallels neurofibrillary tangle formation far more closely than it does amyloid plaque formation. During the earliest definable stage of AD, before symptoms even manifest, amyloid imaging studies performed using PIB-PET show a predominantly frontotemporal pattern (and posterior cingulate) of amyloid deposition, but the only cognitive correlate at this stage is that of modestly accelerated memory decline within the bounds of normal aging (2–4).

Symptomatic disease appears to await neurofibrillary tangle formation, which accompanies synapse loss and neuronal death, and once that begins, specific brain regions are targeted early in its course, especially the cholinergic basal forebrain and medial temporal lobe structures, including the hippocampus, amygdala, and entorhinal cortex (5–8). Because these structures form the neurobiological substrate for memory, severely accelerated memory loss results as an early clinical correlate. AD spreads from there in a characteristic sequence involving posterior cingulate, temporal, and parietal isocortical regions over years. Based on the distribution of these pathological changes, the characteristic "cortical" clinical features of aphasia, apraxia, and agnosia emerge along with consequent amnesia and personality changes.

The NINCDS-ADRDA criteria (Table 5.1) for AD require neuropathological confirmation for a diagnosis of definite Alzheimer's disease (9), and while cortical biopsy can provide a definitive diagnosis during life, this is not routinely performed. Thus, a definitive diagnosis is typically obtained after death.

This does not mean that a clinical diagnosis cannot be made during life. Clinical–pathological correlations rates of 75% in community cohorts (10) and nearly 90% in academic center cohorts (11) have been reported. "Missed" diagnoses are rarely far off (assuming a thorough evaluation as described in Section A has been performed) and more often are attributable to common

Table 5.1 NINCDS-ADRDA Criteria for Probable, Possible, and Definite Alzheimer's Disease

Probable	Dementia established by clinical examination
	Dementia confirmed with cognitive testing
	Deficits in two or more domains of cognition
	Progressive decline of memory and other cognitive functions
	Preserved consciousness
	Onset between ages 40 and 90
	Absence of systemic or other brain disease that account for symptoms
Possible	Atypical onset, presentation, or clinical course of dementia
	Another illness capable of producing dementia is present, but is not considered to be the primary cause
Definite	Clinical criteria for probable AD
	Tissue diagnosis by autopsy or biopsy

McKhann G, Drachman D, Folstein M, et al. Clinical diagnosis of Alzheimer's disease: report of the NINCDS-ADRDA Work Group under the auspices of Department of Health and Human Services Task Force on Alzheimer's Disease. Neurology 1984;34:939–944.

coexisting pathologies, particularly Parkinson's disease and cerebrovascular disease (10,11), warranting an additional or different diagnostic label such as dementia with Lewy bodies, vascular dementia, or another degenerative etiology such as frontotemporal lobar degeneration.

Primarily for research reasons, a succession of neuropathological diagnostic criteria for AD have been established over the past 20 years, with successive refinements, although the basic hallmarks of amyloid plaques and neurofibrillary tangles (Fig. 5.1) have not changed.

The National Institute on Aging established criteria in 1985 that required specific cortical senile plaque densities (12). Cortical neurofibrillary tangles were not required for diagnosis, as some cases of AD were known to be "plaque-only" (13).

The Consortium to Establish a Registry for Alzheimer's Disease (CERAD) published criteria in 1991 (14) that gave diagrammatic semiquantitative standards for assessing plaque density (none, sparse, moderate, or frequent) and specified that only neuritic plaques were relevant for diagnostic purposes, excluding "diffuse" plaques. Diffuse plaques are composed of a 40-amino-acid amyloid fragment felt to be nonpathogenic, and so such plaques do not contain amputated neurites (dendrites and axon fragments from neighboring dead neurons), whereas neuritic plaques are composed of a pathogenic 41- or 42-amino-acid amyloid peptide termed "Aβ" as well as neurites (Fig. 5.2).

The CERAD criteria define Alzheimer's disease once again solely on the basis of cortical plaque density, without a requirement for the presence of cortical neurofibrillary tangles.

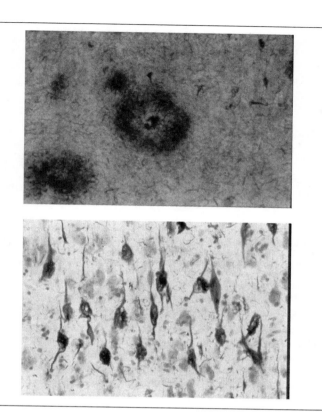

Figure 5.1 Neuropathology of Alzheimer's Disease. Top: neuritic amyloid plaques (Campbell-Switzer stain). Bottom: neurofibrillary tangles (Gallyas stain). Caselli RJ, Beach TG, Yaari R, Reiman EM. Alzheimer's disease a century later. The Journal of Clinical Psychiatry 67(11):1784–800, 2006. Copyright 2006, Physicians Postgraduate Press. Reprinted by permission.

In 1997, a committee formed under the auspices of the National Institute on Aging and the Reagan Institute published new diagnostic criteria that included cortical densities of both neuritic plaques and neurofibrillary tangles (15). These criteria further recognized that more than one factor may contribute to dementia in an elderly patient. Therefore, instead of an all-or-none diagnosis of AD, the Reagan Criteria describe the probability that dementia was due to AD. High cortical densities of both plaques and tangles are designated as "high likelihood that dementia is due to Alzheimer's disease," with lower densities being assigned "intermediate" or "low" likelihoods.

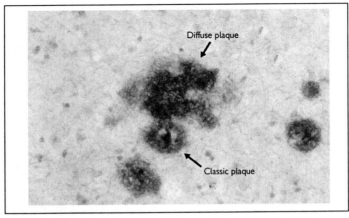

Figure 5.2 Diffuse and neuritic ("classic") plaques side by side in the brain of a patient with Alzheimer's disease. Neuritic plaques are composed of dystrophic neurites containing paired helical filaments of hyperphosphorylated tau that appear as a halo around amyloid cores. Diffuse plaques lack an amyloid core or neuritic halo, may be very irregular in shape, and expand over larger areas of neuropil. Photo courtesy of Dr. Thomas Beach.

An unresolved issue with all these diagnostic criteria is the significance of plaques and tangles in nondemented elderly persons. Current standards restrict the diagnosis of AD to those diagnosed with dementia during life as well as neuropathological evidence at autopsy, but in view of the mounting evidence that genetically at-risk individuals exhibit an accelerated pattern of cognitive aging, this practice may fail to account for many who die during a pre-clinical disease stage.

Pathophysiology

The amyloid plaques and neurofibrillary tangles that are the microscopic signature of AD date back its earliest descriptions, but for many years it was not known whether these were simply nonspecific hallmarks of dead and dying neurons, or actually causing AD. The discovery that early-onset familial AD could be caused by mutations of the amyloid precursor protein (APP) gene on chromosome 21 (16) and the subsequent discoveries of PSEN1 mutations on chromosome 14 (17) and PSEN2 mutations on chromosome 1 (18), each of which cause excess cerebral amyloidosis, made clear that amyloid somehow plays a central role in AD pathogenesis (19–21). (Tau gene mutations also exist but are a cause of frontotemporal lobar degeneration, not AD [22].) However, the exact role that amyloid plays in pathogenesis is still not fully understood. Currently, it is thought that amyloid's role is essentially that of a neuronal toxin.

In both oligomeric and fibrillar plaque form, it kills neurons, and these dead and dying neurons manifest themselves as neurofibrillary tangles and a consequent loss of synapses. Among these pathological features, synaptic loss correlates most closely with clinical measures of dementia severity (23). Amyloid deposition begins early in the course of the disease but, in contrast, correlates poorly with dementia severity. Neurofibrillary tangle formation correlates well with specific deficits such as memory loss (24).

APP is a transmembrane protein, present in all cells (including neurons) on the cell surface and within the endoplasmic reticulum. It is cleaved by three types of proteases, which are designated α-, β- and γ-secretases. In a healthy state, APP is cleaved by α-secretase to form a 40-amino-acid peptide that is soluble or that may contribute to the formation of a benign microscopic lesion, the diffuse plaque. Cleavage by α-secretase destroys the pathogenic Aβ sequence (25). Under conditions of altered energy metabolism due to mitochondrial dysfunction (26), ischemia (27), hypoxia (28), or trauma (29,30) (or other factor), APP is cleaved not by α-secretase, but by β- and γ-secretase releasing Aβ, an insoluble 41- or 42-amino-acid peptide that is pathogenic. β-secretase cleaves APP first to generate a 99-amino-acid membrane-associated fragment (CT99) containing the N-terminus of Aβ peptides (25). γ-secretase then cleaves within the transmembrane region of CT99 to generate the C-terminus of Aβ peptide (25). The production of Aβ peptide is, therefore, dependent on the activities of both β- and γ-secretase.

Monomers and oligomers of abeta have been shown to cause neuronal dysfunction and cognitive impairment in animal models (31). The plaques themselves are formed from deposition of the Aβ fibrillar aggregates. The "amyloid cascade hypothesis" posits that Aβ formation is the primary event leading to AD (19–21) and the cause of all the other relevant but secondary pathological changes, including neurofibrillary tangle formation, loss of synapses, neuronal death, and dementia (Fig. 5.3). Newer models instead propose that the plaques are repositories for the ongoing supply of monomers and oligomers, and that it is these nonaggregated forms that are responsible for Aβ toxicity (32).

The accumulated evidence suggests that plaques occur prior to neurofibrillary tangle formation in neocortical regions and that the latter may possibly form as a neuronal reaction to plaques. Tau is a protein that binds to microtubules, maintaining cytoskeletal integrity. Under disease conditions, it becomes hyperphosphorylated, disaggregates from microtubules, and forms its own paired helical filaments. An alternative theory to the amyloid cascade hypothesis is that phosphorylated forms of tau play the primary role in AD pathogenesis. Support for this theory stems from observations that neuronal microtubules are decreased in AD, and axonal terminals are dependent on them for axoplasmic flow (33). High tangle densities in entorhinal and hippocampal neurons strongly correlate with the memory impairment of normal aging, and much higher tangle densities extending into adjacent medial and inferior temporal cortices correlate with clinically overt AD. In contrast, there is little correlation

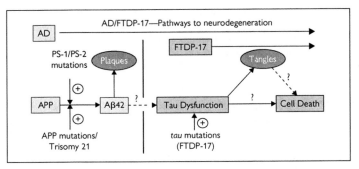

Figure 5.3 The Amyloid Cascade Hypothesis. Genetic alterations that result in increased abeta42/abeta40 ratio enhance plaque deposition, and may also contribute to tau dysfunction and ultimately cell death. Similarly, mutations that result in altered tau metabolism may lead directly to tau hyperphosphorylation and tau pathology. AD=Alzheimer's disease; FTDP-17=Frontotemporal Dementia with Parkinsonism on chromosome 17. (Courtesy of Dr. John Hardy)

between plaque counts or density and dementia severity (34). Further, the earliest neurofibrillary changes in transentorhinal and entorhinal cortex may precede other neuropathology, including abeta deposition (35).

Animal models of AD have generally supported the amyloid hypothesis, as insertion of human APP and PSEN1 gene mutations into transgenic mice result in abeta amyloid plaques that lead to cognitive loss in the absence of tangle formation; tangles themselves do not form unless mutant tau protein genes are also inserted (36).

In summary, AD pathogenesis, in a simplistic way, can be conceived in three major steps, and experimental therapeutic strategies parallel these steps (Fig. 5.4). In step 1, factors such as altered energy metabolism, hypoxia, trauma, or others are deleterious to the brain. Primary prevention strategies are those aimed at step 1 and include measures such as education, antioxidants, and exercise in the hope such interventions might mitigate the impact of these factors. Step 2 is the formation of Aβ amyloid that results from the influence of step 1 factors. Because the bulk of evidence accumulated to date indicates that accumulation of Aβ in the brain is an important step in AD pathogenesis, industry and academic researchers have developed a portfolio of amyloid-modifying treatments, including inhibitors of β-and γ-secretase, anti-aggregation therapies, and active and passive Aβ immunization therapies, which are now in human clinical trials. Aβ production in turn results in step 3, tau hyperphosphorylation, with resultant neuronal death and loss of synapses. There are a smaller number of strategies being considered for the modification of tau pathology.

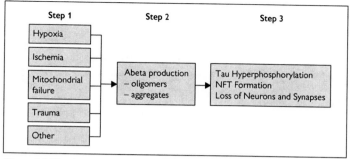

Figure 5.4 The three major pathophysiological stages of Alzheimer's disease are 1) factors that induce an alteration in APP catalysis resulting in 2) the formation of abeta amyloid that in turn leads to 3) tau hyperphosphorylation with neuronal dysfunction and death.

References

1. Bouras C, Hof PR, Giannakopoulos P, et al. Regional distribution of neurofibrillary tangles and senile plaques in the cerebral cortex of elderly patients: a quantitative evaluation of a one-year autopsy population from a geriatric hospital. Cereb Cortex 1994;4:138–150.

2. Klunk WE, Price JC, Mathis CA, et al. Amyloid deposition begins in the striatum of presenilin-1 mutation carriers from two unrelated pedigrees. J Neurosci 2007;27:6174–6184.

3. Reiman EM, Chen K, Liu X, et al. Fibrillar amyloid-beta burden in cognitively normal people at 3 levels of genetic risk for Alzheimer's disease. Proc Natl Acad Sci USA 2009;106:6820–6825.

4. Caselli RJ, Reiman EM, Osborne D, et al. Longitudinal changes in cognition and behavior in asymptomatic carriers of the APOE e4 allele. Neurology 2004;62(11):1990–1995.

5. Braak H, Braak E. Staging of Alzheimer's disease-related neurofibrillary changes. Neurobiol Aging 1995;16:271–278.

6. Braak H, Braak E. Diagnostic criteria for neuropathologic assessment of Alzheimer's disease. Neurobiol Aging 1997;18:S85–S88.

7. Nagy Z, Hindley NJ, Braak H, et al. The progression of Alzheimer's disease from limbic regions to the neocortex: clinical, radiological and pathological relationships. Dement Geriatr Cogn Disord 1999;10:115–120.

8. Beach TG, Kuo YM, Spiegel K, et al. The cholinergic deficit coincides with Abeta deposition at the earliest histopathologic stages of Alzheimer disease. J Neuropathol Exp Neurol 2000;59:308–313.

9. McKhann G, Drachman D, Folstein M, et al. Clinical diagnosis of Alzheimer's disease: report of the NINCDS-ADRDA Work Group under the auspices of Department of Health and Human Services Task Force on Alzheimer's Disease. Neurology 1984;34:939–944.

10. Lim A, Tsuang D, Kukull W, et al. Clinical-neuropathological correlation of Alzheimer's disease in a community-based case series. J Am Geriatr Soc 1999;47:564–569.

11. Klatka LA, Schiffer RB, Powers JM, et al. Incorrect diagnosis of Alzheimer's disease. A clinicopathologic study. Arch Neurol 1996;53:35–42.

12. Khachaturian ZS. Diagnosis of Alzheimer's disease. Arch Neurol 1985;42: 1097–1105.

13. Terry RD, Hansen LA, DeTeresa R, et al. Senile dementia of the Alzheimer type without neocortical neurofibrillary tangles. J Neuropathol Exp Neurol 1987;46:262–268.

14. Mirra SS, Heyman A, McKeel D, et al. The Consortium to Establish a Registry for Alzheimer's Disease (CERAD). Part II. Standardization of the neuropathologic assessment of Alzheimer's disease. Neurology 1991;41:479–486.

15. Hyman BT, Trojanowski JQ. Consensus recommendations for the postmortem diagnosis of Alzheimer disease from the National Institute on Aging and the Reagan Institute Working Group on diagnostic criteria for the neuropathological assessment of Alzheimer disease. J Neuropathol Exp Neurol 1997;56:1095–1097.

16. Goate A, Chartier-Harlin MC, Mullan M, et al. Segregation of a missense mutation in the amyloid precursor protein gene with familial Alzheimer's disease. Nature 1991;349:704–706.

17. Sherrington R, Rogaev EI, Liang Y, et al. Cloning of a gene bearing missense mutations in early-onset familial Alzheimer's disease. Nature 1995;375:754–760.

18. Levy-Lahad E, Wasco W, Poorkaj P, et al. Candidate gene for the chromosome 1 familial Alzheimer's disease locus. Science 1995;269:973–977.

19. Hardy JA, Higgins GA. Alzheimer's disease: the amyloid cascade hypothesis. Science 1992;256:184–185.

20. Neve RL, Robakis NK. Alzheimer's disease: a re-examination of the amyloid hypothesis. Trends Neurosci 1998;21:15–19.

21. Sommer B. Alzheimer's disease and the amyloid cascade hypothesis: ten years on. Curr Opin Pharmacol 2002;2:87–92.

22. Hutton M, Lendon CL, Rizzu P, et al. Association of missense and 5′-splice-site mutations in tau with the inherited dementia FTDP-17. Nature 1998; 393:702–705.

23. Terry RD, Peck A, DeTeresa R, et al. Some morphometric aspects of the brain in senile dementia of the Alzheimer type. Ann Neurol 1981;10:184–192.

24. Hyman BT, Van Hoesen GW, Damasio AR, et al. Alzheimer's disease: cell-specific pathology isolates the hippocampal formation. Science 1984;225:1168–1170.

25. Nunan J, Small DH. Regulation of APP cleavage by alpha-, beta- and gamma-secretases. FEBS Lett 2000;483:6–10.

26. Reddy PH, Beal MF. Are mitochondria critical in the pathogenesis of Alzheimer's disease? Brain Res Rev 2005;49:618–632.

27. Bell RD, Deane R, Chow N, et al. SRF and myocardin regulate LRP-mediated amyloid-B clearance in brain vascular cells. Nature Cell Biol 2009;11:1–11.

28. O'Connor T, Sadleir KR, Maus E, et al. Phosphorylation on the translation initiation factor eIF2a increases BACE1 levels and promotes amyloidogenesis. Neuron 2008;60:988–1009.

29. DeKosky ST, Abrahamson EE, Ciallella JR, et al. Association of increased cortical soluble abeta42 levels with diffuse plaques after severe brain injury in humans. Arch Neurol 2007;64:541–544.

30. Abrahamson EE, Ikonomovic MD, Ciallella JR, et al. Caspase inhibition therapy abolishes brain trauma-induced increases in Abeta peptide: implications for clinical outcome. Exp Neurol 2006;197:437–450.

31. Shankar GM, Bloodgood BL, Townsend M, et al. Natural oligomers of the Alzheimer amyloid-beta protein induce reversible synapse loss by modulating an NMDA-type glutamate receptor-dependent signaling pathway. J Neurosci 2007;27:2866–2875.

32. Selkoe DJ. Soluble oligomers of the amyloid beta-protein impair synaptic plasticity and behavior. Behav Brain Res 2008;192:106–113.

33. Terry RD. The cytoskeleton in Alzheimer disease. J Neural Transm Suppl 1998;53:141–145.

34. Bierer LM, Hof PR, Purohit DP, et al. Neocortical neurofibrillary tangles correlate with dementia severity in Alzheimer's disease. Arch Neurol 1995;52:81–88.

35. Bouras C, Hof PR, Giannakopoulos P, et al. Regional distribution of neurofibrillary tangles and senile plaques in the cerebral cortex of elderly patients: a quantitative evaluation of a one-year autopsy population from a geriatric hospital. Cerebral Cortex 1994;4:138–150.

36. Oddo S, Caccamo A, Shepherd JD, et al. Triple-transgenic model of Alzheimer's disease with plaques and tangles: intracellular abeta and synaptic dysfunction. Neuron 2003;39:409–421.

Chapter 6

The classic clinical syndromes of Alzheimer's disease

Mild Cognitive Impairment

Defining the Clinical Syndrome

Sounding more like a descriptor than a medical diagnosis, mild cognitive impairment (MCI) can be considered an early symptomatic stage when *Diagnostic and Statistical Manual of Mental Disorders, Fourth Edition* (DSM-IV) and National Institute of Neurological and Communicative Disorders and Stroke and the Alzheimer's Disease and Related Disorders Association (NINCDS-ADRDA) criteria for AD have not yet been met, and when diagnostic uncertainty exists. The term "MCI" was originally introduced to define a progressive monosymptomatic amnestic syndrome (1–3) but has since evolved by consensus into an entire classification scheme (Table 6.1) for mild or early-stage, nondisabling cognitive syndromes (4,5).

These constitute amnestic MCI–single domain, amnestic MCI–multiple domains, nonamnestic MCI–single domain, and nonamnestic MCI–multiple domains. Each MCI subtype can then be classified according to the presumed etiology—degenerative, vascular, psychiatric, and so forth. Amnestic MCI, the originally conceived monosymptomatic amnestic form, is often applied to those with a presumed underlying degenerative etiology, particularly AD (Fig. 6.1).

Nonamnestic MCI–single domain refers to monosymptomatic syndromes other than memory loss such as anomia, visual disorders, apraxia, executive disorders, or essentially any deficit that can be considered to be confined to a single cognitive domain. Finally, amnestic and nonamnestic MCI–multiple domain refers to patients with impairment in multiple cognitive domains with and without memory impairment. The defining feature shared by all MCI subtypes is that of an acquired cognitive abnormality that has not yet progressed to the point of causing functional impairment.

MCI and the Conversion Rate to Dementia

The definition and recognition of MCI as an early, if not fully clarified, disease stage is not unique to AD but is nonetheless operationally convenient. MCI can be diagnosed more or less reliably with the help of published criteria (Table 6.1)

Table 6.1 Diagnostic Criteria for Mild Cognitive Impairment

1. General
   a. Symptomatic cognitive complaint
   b. Normal activities of daily living
   c. Normal general cognitive function
   d. Objective cognitive impairment
   e. Does not meet DSM criteria for dementia

2. Single Domain (symptomatic and objective impairment in one of these categories)
   a. Memory
   b. Language
   c. Visuospatial
   d. Executive

3. Multiple Domain (symptomatic and objective impairment in two or more of the above categories)

4. Etiology
   a. Degenerative
   b. Vascular
   c. Other

Winblad B, Palmer K, Kivipelto M, et al. Mild cognitive impairment—beyond controversies, towards a consensus: report of the International Working Group on Mild Cognitive Impairment. J Intern Med 2004; 256: 240–246.

and as patients progress in severity, they eventually cross a diagnostic threshold at which point a diagnosis of AD (or another disorder) becomes appropriate. This is called "conversion" to dementia (or more specifically to AD). The term "conversion" is perhaps misleading as it suggests that something changed, causing a patient who did not have AD to finally succumb to it when, in fact, any patient with MCI who subsequently "converts" to AD already had AD at the MCI stage. MCI is not a risk factor for AD; it *is* AD among those who subsequently "convert." Nonetheless, the MCI and early dementia stages of AD can be distinguished from each other, so the success of interventions aimed at MCI can be measured by the change in "conversion rate" to the early dementia stage of AD (6).

Of its various subtypes, MCI–amnestic is the most specifically correlated with AD (7,8), but it may be less prevalent overall than MCI–multiple cognitive deficits (9). Longitudinal studies of patients with MCI have shown a conversion rate to dementia of roughly 10% to 15% per year (1,2,10,11), although conversion rates vary considerably among studies in part due to different operational definitions of MCI. After 5 years, about half of all patients with MCI will meet the criteria for dementia, particularly AD, and after 10 years, most will have AD or another dementia syndrome. At autopsy, approximately 80% of patients originally diagnosed with MCI prove to have AD (11). Other diagnoses that have been found include vascular dementia, frontotemporal dementia, normal aging, and a variety of less common diseases.

Although MCI has gained widespread acceptance, challenges remain, including but not limited to the absence of a uniform quantitative or systematic definition of functional impairment. The Clinical Dementia Rating Scale (12) has been used

Amnestic MCI

Orientation	7/8
Attention	7/7
Learning	4/4
Arithmetic	4/4
Constructions	4/4
Abstractions	3/3
Information	4/4
Recall	0/4
Total	33/38

Letter (or Cartegory) Fluency: unimpaired
Naming: unimpaired
Writing: unimapaired
Simultanagnosia? No
Familiar Faces: unimpaired
History: Memory loss
Physical: unimpaired

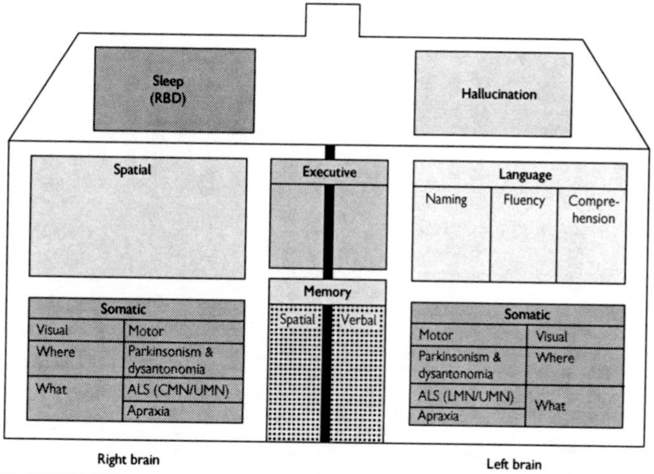

Figure 6.1 Amnestic MCI. History and mental status testing reflect relatively isolated memory difficulties including both verbal and spatial aspects of memory.

in research studies and has proven to be a valuable instrument for the definition of functional impairment. It is too time-consuming, however, for practical clinical application. Because of the relatively recent definition of MCI subtypes, their differences from one another continue to be clarified, including their incidence, prevalence, neuropathological correlates, and rates of conversion to AD.

Alzheimer's Dementia

Syndromes

MCI is one example of a clinical syndrome caused by AD. In many patients it happens to be an early stage of AD, but even in these cases it is termed MCI to distinguish it from the more complete syndrome that characterizes the dementia stages of AD. Dementing illnesses tend to produce characteristic profiles of cognitive symptoms and signs, and recognizing these distinctive profiles greatly aids in clinical diagnosis. A patient has AD first and foremost because he or she has the clinical appearance of AD. AD is not simply a diagnosis of exclusion, even if much of the supporting evidence is exclusionary. This is a simple but important concept when considering alternative and potentially reversible diagnoses. Reversible diseases (such as those associated with an infectious, inflammatory, toxic, or metabolic cause) do not generally reproduce the specific pattern of cognitive deficits that define AD, but one can appreciate and recognize that only if one knows what AD looks like. When a patient's cognitive profile fails to fall into a recognizable degenerative category, particular care should be taken to exclude a potentially reversible cause.

Alzheimer's *disease* is a pathologically defined disease process that typically results in a characteristic pattern of cognitive deficits that may be termed Alzheimer's *dementia*. Alzheimer's *dementia* is characterized by prominent memory loss, anomia, constructional apraxia (Fig. 6.2), anosognosia, and variable degrees of personality change in which patients can become mistrustful and aggressive, or frankly delusional and belligerent (13).

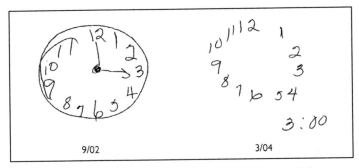

9/02   3/04

Figure 6.2 Constructional apraxia developing in a patient with Alzheimer's disease as illustrated by a clock drawing task.

Alzheimer's *disease* does not always produce this pattern, however. Visual variant AD, or posterior cortical atrophy, is a syndrome in which patients develop progressive visual impairment related to atypically early and severe degenerative involvement of posterior visual cortices (14). Other focal variants of AD are less common but include progressive aphasia (typically fluent aphasia), progressive apraxia, and progressive frontotemporal dementia (15–18). Anecdotally, the more posterior AD variants, such as visual variant and apraxic forms, may be less prone to behavioral difficulties than the typical and more anterior (aphasic and frontotemporal) forms.

Two commonly used sets of criteria for the diagnosis of AD are those of the 1984 NINCDS-ADRDA joint task force (Table 6.2) (19) and DSM-IV (Table 6.3) (20).

Table 6.2 NINCDS-ADRDA Criteria for Probable, Possible, and Definite Alzheimer's Disease

Probable	Dementia established by clinical examination
	Dementia confirmed with cognitive testing
	Deficits in two or more domains of cognition
	Progressive decline of memory and other cognitive functions
	Preserved consciousness
	Onset between ages 40 and 90
	Absence of systemic or other brain disease that account for symptoms
Possible	Atypical onset, presentation, or clinical course of dementia
	Another illness capable of producing dementia is present, but is not considered to be the primary cause
Definite	Clinical criteria for probable AD
	Tissue diagnosis by autopsy or biopsy

Table 6.3 DSM-IV-TR Criteria for Dementia of the Alzheimer's Type

Insidious onset with progressive decline of cognitive function resulting in impairment of social or occupational functioning from a previously higher level
Impairment of recent memory
Disturbance in at least one of the following cognitive domains: • Aphasia   • Apraxia   • Agnosia   • Executive functioning (planning, organizing, sequencing, abstracting)
Cognitive deficits are not due to other neurologic, psychiatric, toxic, metabolic, or systemic diseases
Cognitive deficits do not occur solely in the setting of a delirium

Criteria for probable AD include dementia with cognitive deficits in at least two cognitive domains including progressive memory loss (Fig. 6.3), normal level of consciousness, onset between ages 40 and 90 years, and the absence of another plausible medical explanation. If there is another illness that might be contributing to the clinical picture but is not felt to be the primary cause of dementia, or if the picture is dominated by a progressive focal cognitive deficit (e.g., progressive aphasia), then the term "possible Alzheimer's disease" is used. The diagnosis of definite AD requires the neuropathological diagnosis of AD (typically at autopsy, but sometimes from a brain tissue biopsy).

DSM-IV criteria for dementia of the Alzheimer's type (see Table 6.3) include a gradual and progressive decline in cognitive function resulting in impairment of social or occupational function and an impairment in recent memory and at least one other cognitive domain (aphasia, apraxia, agnosia, or executive functioning) that are not due to other psychiatric or nonpsychiatric medical problems. Since neuropathological confirmation is not required, DSM-IV criteria for dementia of the Alzheimer's type most closely resemble NINCDS-ADRA criteria for probable AD.

Stages of Clinical Severity

Staging clinical severity in AD patients is an imprecise exercise, although functional staging systems such as the Clinical Dementia Rating (CDR) scale (12) are helpful in research settings. The CDR grades each of six functional domains that in turn can serve as a guide for clinicians in their attempts to assess functional impairment: memory, orientation, judgment and problem solving, community affairs, home and hobbies, and personal care. The CDR uses a scale from 0 (no impairment) to 3 (severe impairment) to generate an overall functional score. Because of its prevalence in the literature, it is useful for clinicians to at least be aware of CDR classification schemes. CDR scoring rules result in categorizing a patient as normal (CDR = 0) or having MCI (CDR = 0.5), mild dementia (CDR = 1), moderate dementia (CDR = 2), or severe dementia (CDR = 3). Higher scores imply greater patient needs and caregiver burden. Behavioral and sleep issues pose the greatest caregiver burden, generally more so than intellectual impairment (e.g., memory loss). In patients with highly discrepant levels of impairment in different symptomatic categories, it can be difficult to stage the disease. For example, if a patient with mild dementia develops the paranoid delusion that his wife is cheating on him and assaults her as a result, his problem is severe even if his degree of intellectual decline is mild. Conversely, a patient with aphasic variant AD who is completely unable to communicate may still be able to dress, act in a socially appropriate way, and maintain his or her own hygiene. The language impairment is severe, but he or she would be less of a burden to a caregiver than the first example. With these very real limitations in mind, the following descriptions offer a rough staging guideline for clinicians.

Mild Stage

Most clinical studies agree that the earliest clinical sign of AD is memory loss. Recent memory is more reliably assessed than remote memory and is thought

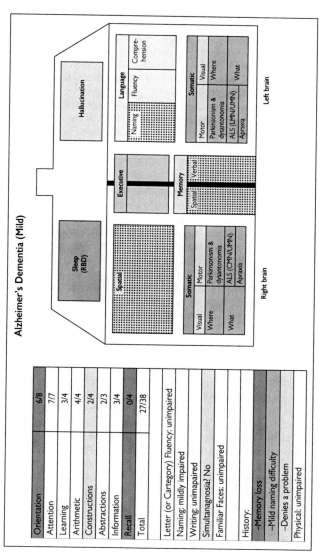

Orientation	6/8
Attention	7/7
Learning	3/4
Arithmetic	4/4
Constructions	2/4
Abstractions	2/3
Information	3/4
Recall	0/4
Total	27/38

Letter (or Cartegory) Fluency: unimpaired

Naming: mildly impaired

Writing: unimapaired

Simultanagnosia? No

Familiar Faces: unimpaired

History:
  –Memory loss
  –Mild naming difficulty
  –Denies a problem

Physical: unimpaired

Figure 6.3 Alzheimer's Dementia. Two or more cognitive domains, one of which is memory, are impaired. As illustrated here, spatial and language impairment (anomia) are very common, and patients often deny they have a problem.

to be disproportionately severely impaired. Nonetheless, remote memory may also be abnormal. There is a gradient effect for recall over a retrograde time interval: the oldest memories are the best preserved, with proportionately greater forgetting as the retrograde interval shortens. In contrast, procedural memory appears to be spared in early stages. AD patients are able to learn simple skills as easily as normal controls and better than patients with subcortical patterns of dementia and patients with various types of sensorimotor deficits (21,22). This may explain the observations of patients and families that skills such as playing a musical instrument, riding a bicycle, or even driving seem relatively unimpaired during early-stage disease. With regard to driving, however, despite the relative preservation of procedural memory, patients with mild Alzheimer's dementia have a higher rate of collisions and moving violations than age-matched controls (23), although estimates of risk vary, especially during the first 2 years of the disease. Whether this actually results from impaired procedural memory, attentional factors, other cognitive aspects, or a combination is unclear.

Moderate Stage

Aphasia, apraxia, and agnosia characterize this stage of AD. In mild to moderate stages of dementia, anomia is prominent and readily detectable with neuro-psychological testing. Patients are fluent and may have relatively good comprehension, so clinical detection is not always easy. As the disease progresses, the predominantly anomic aphasia gives way to a more fluent, or Wernicke's, type of aphasia with impaired comprehension. Although apraxia is one of the defining features of cortical dementia, it is rarely severe in mild to moderate stages of AD and can be very difficult to distinguish from impaired comprehension in these patients. Patients have difficulty performing tasks at which they were previously adept, such as repairing a household appliance or doing carpentry work. They also have difficulty learning new procedures such as operating a new car, new appliance, or remote control device. They have some difficulty pantomiming gestures in the office setting but also have constructional apraxia. In moderately advanced stages, patients have trouble dressing and performing other activities of daily living. Patients with clinically evident apraxia typically also have significant perceptual difficulties. Anosognosia, the failure to recognize illness, is a cardinal feature of Alzheimer's dementia. It may be present even in mild stages of the disease. Typical patients with anosognosia are brought or sent for evaluation rather than coming of their own accord, and actively try to explain away the observations of concerned family members and friends, even to the point of becoming hostile and accusative. Other agnosic disturbances in these patients include occasionally failing to recognize someone familiar, such as a friend or other acquaintance, and difficulty learning their way around a once-familiar home (such as their children's) or neighborhood.

Severe Stage

Language deficits progress to the point of a disabling fluent aphasia, and it may be difficult to understand what the patient is trying to relate. Apraxia progresses to the point of impairing activities of daily living such as dressing, eating, and maintaining personal hygiene. In moderate to advanced stages, patients

exhibit other agnosic types of disturbances. Their difficulty in recognizing familiar people (prosopagnosia) now affects family members, even spouses. Unlike true prosopagnosics, AD patients are not reliably benefited by voice recognition. Difficulty finding their way worsens and could be compared with topographagnosia, another visual agnosic syndrome. Simultanagnosia is an inability to view all parts of a complex visual scene in a single coherent time–space frame. Such patients fail to see a target object that is right in front of them, especially if it is surrounded by potentially distracting stray objects (14). Strictly speaking, this is not an agnosic disorder but another type of complex visual disturbance that resembles agnosia and can occur in this setting. Reduplicative paramnesia or Capgras syndrome is the delusional belief that a spouse (or other significant person) is an imposter, or that there are "two Julia's." Also, home may not be recognized as home, and some other place is believed to exist that is the real home.

Incontinence (both urinary and fecal) is uncommon in mild stages, becomes increasingly frequent as the disease progresses, and is nearly universal in late stages. Early on, it may inadvertently result from voiding in the "wrong place" rather than actual loss of sphincter control, but in later stages, sphincter control is lost. Weight loss is common during the severe stage as well.

Terminal Stage

Preterminal- and terminal-stage AD ensues after roughly a 5- to 10-year course of overt cognitive impairment, but this is highly variable and depends greatly on when the disease is considered to begin. In very advanced stages, patients are no longer ambulatory, become mute and incontinent, and are totally dependent on a caregiver. Death can result from urosepsis, pulmonary embolism, or other intercurrent illnesses. Few patients live to these latter stages, but for those who do, behavioral output declines so that patients do less of everything. They talk less and are less active or even bedbound. It becomes impossible to accurately assess their perceptual abilities, although they are probably also severely impaired. Ultimately swallowing and balance difficulties arise and choking, aspiration, and falls occur that can ultimately lead to death.

Behavioral Symptoms

Psychiatric symptoms can emerge at any stage from MCI to severe but are very common in the moderate and severe stages. These include both affective and psychotic disturbances. Depression can also be erroneously diagnosed as dementia (pseudodementia) since it impairs functional status, and depressed patients often fail to perform accurately on cognitive assessments. Pseudodementia has been estimated to account for 4% to 5% of dementia cases (24). More commonly, however, depression may complicate the course of AD and other dementias. Psychotic symptoms most commonly involve paranoid delusions and, less commonly, hallucinations (visual hallucinations, in contrast, are a hallmark of dementia with Lewy bodies). Rarely paranoid delusions may be a presenting feature, and AD should be considered in any elderly patient presenting de novo with a delusional syndrome or hallucinosis. Common paranoid themes involve infidelity and theft. Hallucinations are generally complex, involving people (familiar or unfamiliar), animals, or both. The combination of anosognosia, paranoid delusions, and mild cognitive decline is a recipe for potentially dangerous behavior and is very difficult to manage, especially if such individuals live alone, yet a significant minority of AD patients have exactly that combination.

Sleep–wake cycle disturbances are common and may be present even during relatively mild stages of the illness. They become more common and more severe during later stages. There are two aspects to the sleep–wake cycle disturbance. The first is the so-called sundowning effect, which means that the patient becomes more confused, agitated, and difficult to manage during the evening hours. The second regards either not sleeping at night, waking up during very early hours, or going to sleep very early in the evening. Sleep becomes fractionated into shorter segments throughout the 24-hour period. As the disease progresses to more advanced stages, patients may become generally less active, sleep more, and eventually, in terminal stages, are bedbound with little activity.

References

1. Petersen RC, Smith GE, Ivnik RJ, et al. Apolipoprotein E status as a predictor of the development of Alzheimer's disease in memory-impaired individuals. JAMA 1995;273:1274–1278.

2. Petersen RC, Smith GE, Waring SC, et al. Mild cognitive impairment: clinical characterization and outcome. Arch Neurol 1999;56:303–308.

3. Petersen RC, Stevens JC, Ganguli M, et al. Practice parameter: early detection of dementia: mild cognitive impairment (an evidence-based review). Report of the Quality Standards Subcommittee of the American Academy of Neurology. Neurology 2001;56:1133–1142.

4. Petersen RC, Doody R, Kurz A, et al. Current concepts in mild cognitive impairment. Arch Neurol 2001;58:1985–1992.

5. Winblad B, Palmer K, Kivipelto M, et al. Mild cognitive impairment—beyond controversies, towards a consensus: report of the International Working Group on Mild Cognitive Impairment. J Intern Med 2004;256:240–246.

6. Petersen RC, Thomas RG, Grundman M, et al. Vitamin E and donepezil for the treatment of mild cognitive impairment. N Engl J Med 2005;352:2379–2388.

7. Busse A, Bischkopf J, Riedel-Heller SG, et al. Subclassifications for mild cognitive impairment: prevalence and predictive validity. Psychol Med 2003;33:1029–1038.

8. Rasquin SM, Lodder J, Visser PJ, et al. Predictive accuracy of MCI subtypes for Alzheimer's disease and vascular dementia in subjects with mild cognitive impairment: a 2-year follow-up study. Dement Geriatr Cogn Disord 2005;19:113–119.

9. Lopez OL, Jagust WJ, DeKosky ST, et al. Prevalence and classification of mild cognitive impairment in the Cardiovascular Health Study Cognition Study: part 1. Arch Neurol 2003;60:1385–1389.

10. Ganguli M, Dodge HH, Shen C, et al. Mild cognitive impairment, amnestic type: an epidemiologic study. Neurology 2004;63:115–121.

11. Morris JC, Storandt M, Miller JP, et al. Mild cognitive impairment represents early-stage Alzheimer disease. Arch Neurol 2001;58:397–405.

12. Morris JC, Ernesto C, Schafer K, et al. Clinical dementia rating training and reliability in multicenter studies: the Alzheimer's Disease Cooperative Study experience. Neurology 1997;48:1508–1510.

13. Rossor MN. Primary degenerative dementia. In Bradley WG, Daroff RB, Fenichel GM, et al, eds. Neurology in Clinical Practice, 2nd ed. Boston: Butterworth-Heinemann, 1996:1586–1599.

14. Tang-Wai DF, Graff-Radford NR, Boeve BF, et al. Clinical, genetic, and neuropathologic characteristics of posterior cortical atrophy. Neurology 2004;63:1168–1174.

15. Caselli RJ, Jack CR, Jr. Asymmetric cortical degeneration syndromes. A proposed clinical classification. Arch Neurol 1992;49:770–780

16. Caselli RJ, Stelmach GE, Caviness JN, et al. A kinematic study of progressive apraxia with and without dementia. Mov Disord 1999;14:276–287.

17. Johnson JK, Head E, Kim R, et al. Clinical and pathological evidence for a frontal variant of Alzheimer disease. Arch Neurol 1999;56:1233–1239.

18. Boeve BF, Maraganore DM, Parisi JE, et al. Pathologic heterogeneity in clinically diagnosed corticobasal degeneration. Neurology 1999;53:795–800.

19. McKhann G, Drachman D, Folstein M, et al. Clinical diagnosis of Alzheimer's disease: report of the NINCDS-ADRDA Work Group under the auspices of Department of Health and Human Services Task Force on Alzheimer's Disease. Neurology 1984;34:939–944.

20. American Psychiatric Association. Desk Reference to the Diagnostic Criteria from DSM-IV. Washington DC: APA, 1994:85.

21. Beatty WW, Salmon DP, Butters N, et al. Retrograde amnesia in patients with Alzheimer's or Huntington's disease. Neurobiol Aging 1988;9:181–186.

22. Heindel WC, Salmon DP, Shults CW, et al. Neuropsychological evidence for multiple memory systems: a comparison of Alzheimer's, Huntington's, and Parkinson's disease patients. J Neurosci 1989;9:582–587.

23. Fitten LJ, Perryman KM, Wilkinson CJ, et al. Alzheimer and vascular dementias and driving: a prospective road and laboratory study. JAMA 1995;273:1360–1365.

24. Clarfield AM. The reversible dementias: do they reverse? Ann Intern Med 1988;109:476–486.

Chapter 7

Clinical variants of Alzheimer's disease

General Principles of Neurodegenerative Topography and the Origin of Clinical "Variants"

AD can follow more than one symptomatic trajectory. The most common trajectory is that which we have just considered: initial memory loss that becomes severe early as the additional deficits of aphasia, apraxia, and agnosia begin to unfold in balanced proportion with or without additional psychiatric and other features continuously worsening in severity until a late stage of severe impairment encompassing all domains and producing complete functional disability. Although memory loss is a nearly obligate early-stage symptom, AD can follow some very different symptomatic trajectories. Fortunately for diagnostic purposes, most such variants are not very subtle, but instead tend to dominate a particular cognitive domain, so that rather than a balance between aphasia, apraxia, and agnosia, one evolves early and much more severely than the other two, sometimes leading to the premature and erroneous diagnosis of stroke. Because this "lopsided" presentation reflects disproportionate involvement of one side or region of the brain, these can be considered focal variants or, more correctly, "asymmetrical cortical degeneration syndromes" (1–5) (Fig. 7.1).

These can occur as variants of AD but in some cases represent the more typical presentation of a different (and less common) degenerative disease.

Underlying each of the focal variant syndromes is a shared topographical principle illustrated in Fig. 7.2. This pair of monozygotic twins was phenotypically discordant for the syndrome of progressive apraxia. There is a gradient of pathology as reflected by cerebral metabolism and atrophy. Topographically, the most severely hypometabolic and atrophic region is also the most symptomatic area. In the example shown, the proband presented with a visuomotor syndrome. He was unable to visually locate objects embedded in a complex visual scene and developed progressive apraxia affecting the left much more than the right upper limb. Speech, however, was (relatively) unimpaired. Corresponding to this clinical pattern of impairment, we see that his most severely hypometabolic and atrophic cerebral region is the right parietotemporal junction. This therefore represents the primary degenerative focus. The

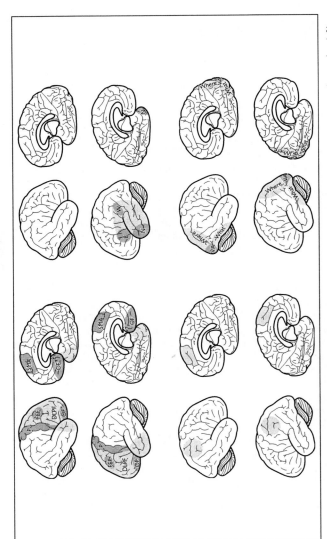

Figure 7.1 Topographical-clinical patterns of asymmetric cortical degeneration include frontotemporal dysexecutive syndromes (top left), progressive aphasia (top right), progressive apraxia (bottom left), and progressive visual syndrome (bottom right). Caselli RJ. Asymmetric cortical degeneration: syndromes and diseases. Neurologist 1995;1:1–20.

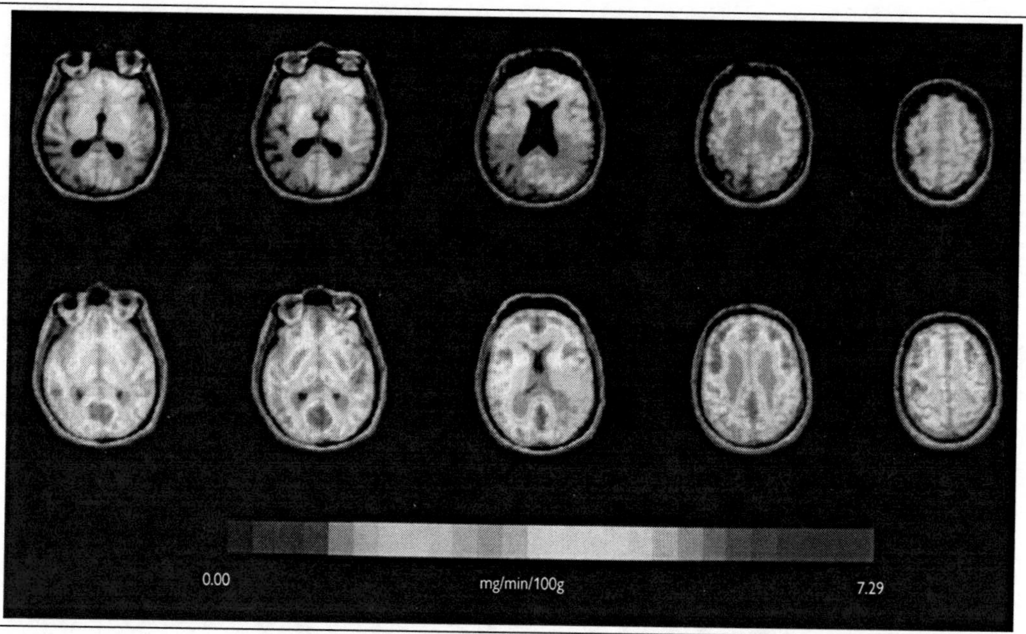

Figure 7.2 Progressive apraxia in clinically discordant monozygotic twins. The top row is the proband, and the bottom row his asymptomatic twin brother. See text for details. Caselli RJ, Reiman EM, Timmann D, Stelmach GE, Lawson MA, Osborne D, Moore SB, Cevette MJ. Progressive apraxia in clinically discordant monozygotic twins. Arch Neurol. Oct 1995, 52(10):1004–10. Copyright (1995) American Medical Association. All Rights Reserved.

contralateral homologous cerebral region is the next most severely affected region, constituting the secondary degenerative focus. Note that stroke patients' recovery relies upon contiguous and contralateral regions, whereas in the degenerative context, contiguous and contralateral regions are also involved, perhaps impeding their chances for recovery.

Finally, a comparison of the proband to his identical twin shows there is a more generalized or tertiary level of degeneration. Compare, for example, the prefrontal regions. This area is relatively spared when compared to the parietal and temporal cortices within the patient's own brain, but when we compare the prefrontal cortices to the unaffected twin there is a clear difference. Also, the relative general atrophy of the proband's brain is easily seen when comparing ventricular size with the unaffected twin. (Incidentally noted as well is reduced metabolism in the left parietotemporal region of the twin, raising the possibility that the pair are actually concordant but that other unidentified factors are preventing symptomatic expression in the asymptomatic twin.)

Thus, we see that in a focal variant there is a hierarchy of degenerative topography. The clinical syndrome reflects the primary area of involvement, but there is also a secondary contralateral area of involvement contributing the severity of the disorder, and a more generalized tertiary level of involvement. Comparing cognitive skills referable to each of these three levels of involvement shows that when compared to an identical and unaffected twin, these areas are all dysfunctional, albeit to a lesser degree than the primary degenerative focus. Although the example illustrated is one of progressive apraxia, this pattern is applicable to each of the focal variants. Finally, typical AD is characterized by a pattern of relatively symmetrical, bilateral parietal and temporal (among other areas) hypometabolism. The asymmetrical variants exaggerate this pattern in a laterally unbalanced way so that we see right hemisphere and left hemisphere syndromes emerge, as well as more posterior and more anterior syndromes, as we shall now discuss.

Asymmetrical Cortical Degeneration Syndromes: Visual Variants

Visual Syndromes

Visual variant AD is also called "posterior cortical atrophy" based upon the generally prominent and disproportionate degree of atrophy that can be seen on structural imaging studies in the occipitoparietal and, to a lesser degree, occipitotemporal cortices. Progressive visual syndromes involve degeneration of parieto-occipital and/or parieto-temporal visual association cortices. Visual association cortices can be broadly divided into dorsal (occipitoparietal) and ventral (occipitotemporal) pathways, and disorders of visual association cortices will reflect this dichotomy (Fig. 7.3).

The occipitoparietal pathways map space and link search strategies (eye movements and reaching movements) to that spatial map allowing us to locate

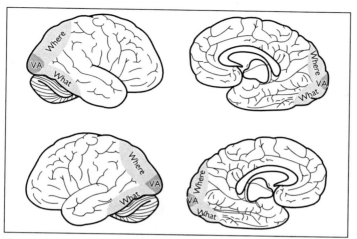

Figure 7.3 Progressive visual syndromes are also termed "visual variant Alzheimer's disease" and "posterior cortical atrophy" and are characterized by dysfunction of the "where and what" pathways. Occipitoparietal (where) degeneration most often results from Alzheimer's disease, but occipitotemporal (or more anteriorly situated right temporal degeneration) may reflect frontotemporal lobar degeneration. Caselli RJ. Asymmetric cortical degeneration: syndromes and diseases. Neurologist 1995;1:1–20.

and retrieve an object ("where") of interest. The occipitotemporal pathways instead are concerned with object identification ("what") and the disambiguation of visually similar exemplars within the same object category (e.g., distinguishing faces). Two broadly defined types of complex visual disturbance can result from AD that reflect this functional dichotomy (6).

Asimultanagnosia

The first and more commonly reported is progressive asimultanagnosia (the inability to compute simultaneity); it results from degeneration of occipitoparietal cortices (Fig. 7.4) (7,8).

As we visually scan a scene, we are taking multiple snapshots that our brain must fuse together into a single coherent time–space reference frame. All those visual bits coexist at a single point in time as part of a single integrated spatial scene. Patients with asimultanagnosia cannot perform this function and consequently fail to see things that may be right in front of them (Fig. 7.5). They are at an extreme disadvantage when trying to search for an object given their lack of a coherent spatial reference frame. Asimultanagnosia was first described as a central component of "Balint's syndrome" (the other components of Balint's involve the secondary consequences of impaired eye and limb search movements) that resulted from bilateral parietal lesions (9). Balint's syndrome was initially thought to reflect a psychiatric disorder ("psychic blindness") because when tested with conventional eye charts, patients' visual acuity was

Posterior Cortical Atrophy (Visual Variant Alzheimer's Disease)

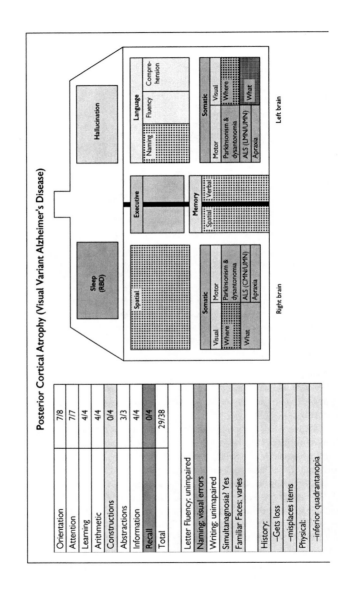

Orientation	7/8
Attention	7/7
Learning	4/4
Arithmetic	4/4
Constructions	0/4
Abstractions	3/3
Information	4/4
Recall	0/4
Total	29/38

Letter Fluency: unimpaired

Naming: visual errors

Writing: unimapaired

Simultanagnosia? Yes

Familiar Faces: varies

History:
–Gets loss
–misplaces items

Physical:
–inferior quadrantanopia

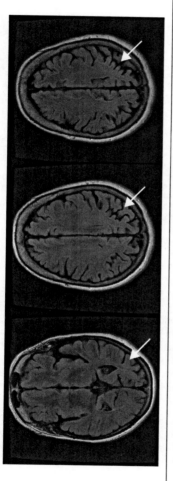

Figure 7.4 Visual Variant Alzheimer's Disease in a 64 year old woman. Visual impairment manifests as simultanagnosia ("where") and moreso than prosopagnosia ("what"). Naming objects may seem impaired if they are not adequately visualized. Constructional ability and memory is usually impaired as well. Note the asymmetric atrophy that is most pronounced in the left occipitoparietal, and to some extent occipitotemporal cortices.

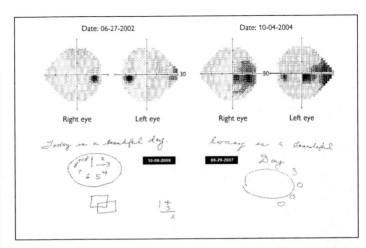

Figure 7.5 Visual field (top row) and constructional praxis between ages 64 and 68 years in a woman with visual variant Alzheimer's disease. Folstein MMSE declined from 30 in 2002 to 14 in 2007 in parallel with her progressive left hemianopia and constructional apraxia. Although her visual field deficit may appear mild on these charts, she was unable to find objects as large as a soup ladle or ash tray that were placed in front of her in plain sight when they were in a container cluttered with other objects (asimultanagnosia).

unimpaired, and responses on visual field tests were highly inconsistent, as can be found in some psychiatric patients.

Because degenerative diseases rarely respect strict topographical or functional boundaries, a variety of other disturbances may occur in these patients that also reflect the functions of posterior cortices. Memory loss, a near-universal feature of patients with any form of AD, seems less severe relative to the visual disturbance in this subset of patients, at least during mild to moderate stages of the disease, and other deficits include alexia, acalculia, right–left disorientation, and mild comprehension deficits (fluent aphasia). Some patients may be found to have an inferior quadrantanopia (7,8).

Prosopagnosia

Figure 7.6 is an MRI of a patient's brain showing striking right (greater than left bilateral) anterior temporal atrophy. This pattern of atrophy is more characteristic of a subtype of frontotemporal lobar degeneration (FTLD) than of AD (10,11). (We will consider the left temporal lobe version of this disorder, semantic dementia, with the aphasia variants.)

Generally, FTLD patients are younger, so that such a pattern in a 60-year-old is more likely to be FTLD, but such a pattern in an 80-year-old may in fact reflect an AD variant. The occipitotemporal visual pathway terminates in the anterior temporal lobes and subserves specific object recognition, particularly

Prosopagnosic Semantic Dementia (right > left temporal atrophy)

Orientation	8/8
Attention	7/7
Learning	4/4
Arithmetic	4/4
Constructions	4/4
Abstractions	2/3
Information	4/4
Recall	3/4
Total	36/38

Letter (or Cartegory) Fluency: unimpaired

Naming: mildly impaired

Writing: unimpaired

Simultanagnosia? No

Familiar Faces: unimpaired

History:
- Less active
- Failure to recognize familiar people
- May get lost easily

Physical:
MRI striking right temporal atrophy

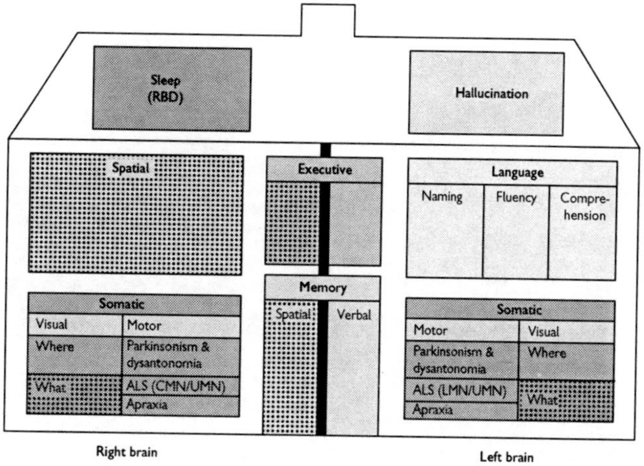

Figure 7.6 Right greater than left bitemporal atrophy in a 77 year old man with a two year history of progressive facial recognition difficulties (the "what" pathway), memory loss, and personality changes.

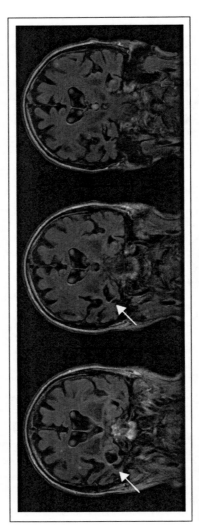

Figure 7.6 *Continued.*

that aspect involved in the disambiguation of visually similar objects. Faces are a socially important category of object, and our brains may have evolved specialized systems for facial disambiguation and recognition above and beyond our ability to disambiguate, for example, bananas. Consequently, patients with this pattern of degeneration have impaired ability to distinguish familiar faces, a visual syndrome called "prosopagnosia." This can be quite subtle in early stages, but a test of famous faces (for example, past presidents and movie stars) can readily detect the problem (12). Unfortunately, such tests of famous faces are not routinely performed in either the physician's office or even in most neuropsychology laboratories unless the specific question is highlighted. Nonetheless, a small collection of 5 or 10 very famous faces taken from magazines and the Internet (or family photographs) can be sufficient to demonstrate the problem in many cases. Impaired facial recognition plus the MRI appearance shown essentially defines the syndrome of progressive prosopagnosia. Such patients again have memory difficulties or anomia, and some may have alexia due to left temporal lobe involvement, but that is the exception rather than the rule. Bilateral temporal atrophy can also cause personality changes that range from passivity to hyperactivity; the reason for such differences may reflect the specific subregions of the temporal and frontal cortices affected that vary between individual patients.

Asymmetrical Cortical Degeneration Syndromes: Aphasic Variants

Though original credit belongs to Arnold Pick for correlating lobar atrophy with aphasic dementia (13), Mesulam's 1982 report of progressive aphasia (14) essentially refocused modern neurology on the relationship of focal cortical degeneration to a progressive cortical syndrome. Because most patients are left hemisphere dominant for language, most patients have left-sided asymmetrical atrophy. However, occasional patients are found who are left-handed and who have right hemisphere asymmetrical atrophy accompanying progressive aphasia. Cognitive deficits other than those directly attributable to language may also occur, especially memory impairment and constructional apraxia. Although theoretically every conceivable subtype of aphasia can be seen, there are four predominant aphasic variants in AD patients (Fig. 7.7).

Fluent Aphasia

This is the most common of the aphasic variants in AD patients and reflects degeneration of temporal and posterior temporoparietal perisylvian cortices (Fig. 7.8) (15).

Contiguous involvement of neighboring cortices may complicate the clinical picture, making it difficult to distinguish a focal left temporoparietal syndrome (with aphasia, amnesia, apraxia, and acalculia) from a "diffuse" cognitive disorder. Fluency, articulation, and prosody (the melody or expressivity of speech) are normal, but comprehension and naming are impaired. Word, number, and sentence repetition appears to be impaired less consistently in early stages but is usually impaired with further clinical progression. Number

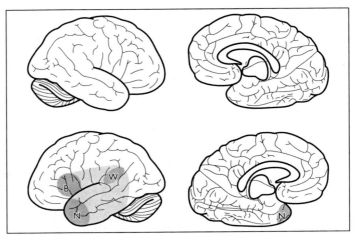

Figure 7.7 Progressive aphasic sydromes reflect perisylvian atrophy of the language dominant (usually left) hemisphere. The four predominant patterns discernible in the context of degenerative dementia are fluent, nonfluent, anomic (also called semantic dementia), and mixed. Fluent and mixed ae usually caused by Alzheimer's disease whereas nonfluent and anomic may result from frontotemporal lobar degeneration. Caselli RJ. Asymmetric cortical degeneration: syndromes and diseases. Neurologist 1995;1:1–20.

repetition or digit span is sometimes considered an attention-based skill and so impairment might be interpreted a sign of executive dysfunction, but in the context of aphasia it is more likely a language-based error. When trying to name an object, for example a wrench, a generic descriptor such as "tool" or an intracategorical error such as "pliers" may be spoken instead. Such errors are called semantic paraphasias. (In contrast, patients with nonfluent aphasia will say phonemic paraphasias that are sound substitutions within the correct target word, such as "wrenk.") Alternatively, a patient may simply describe the object or demonstrate its use in trying to name it ("something I use…"). The language deficit that evolves in patients with typical AD is also fluent, but aphasic variant patients have disproportionately more severe language impairment at an earlier stage with relative sparing of other domains, including spatial and social skills and insight.

Nonfluent Aphasia

Figure 7.9 is an MRI of a patient's brain showing left frontal opercular atrophy that corresponds to Broca's area. This pattern of atrophy is more characteristic of a subtype of FTLD called "primary progressive nonfluent aphasia" than of AD, but it can occur in either (16).

Among patients with nonfluent aphasia due to FTLD, a small subset develop motor neuron disease, making recognition of this syndrome particularly

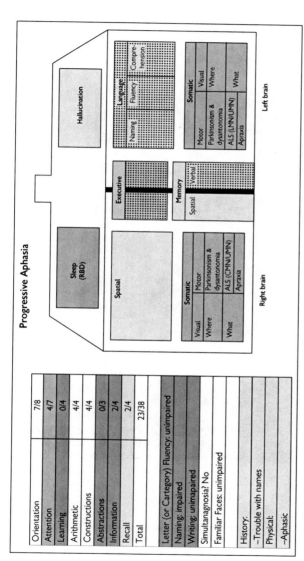

Figure 7.8 Fluent aphasia with extensive left hemisphere atrophy including temporal and parietal cortices in a 72 year old woman with a several year history of progressive naming and comprehension difficulties. Note that verbal memory and executive skills are also often impaired, though to varying degrees. Many tests for executive skills, such as digit span, rely upon language and so may be secondarily impaired as a result of the aphasia.

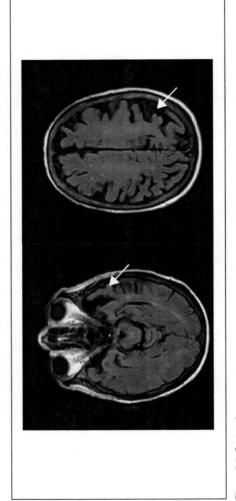

Figure 7.8 *Continued.*

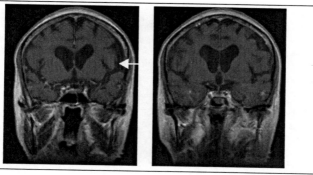

Figure 7.9 Progressive nonfluent aphasia with left frontal opercular atrophy in a 74 year old woman with a 4 year history of slowly progressive word finding difficulty with increasingly effortful speech.

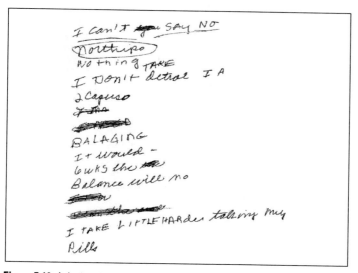

Figure 7.10 Aphasic written comments of a 74 year old woman with aphasic variant Alzheimer's disease.

important, but there is no similar association with motor neuron disease in AD patients. Speech is effortful, halting, and sometimes apraxic or dysarthric. Naming ability is marked by phonemic paraphasic errors in which sound substitutions are made within the correct target word (for example, "captus" for cactus). Sentence repetition is generally severely impaired, and writing is sometimes easier than speaking, although usually still abnormal (Fig. 7.10).

Aural and reading comprehension are less impaired in mild to moderate stages, but they deteriorate in most with disease progression. Some patients have orofacial apraxia (e.g., they may have trouble blowing out a candle) but not gestural or limb apraxia. Verbal memory tests are difficult to administer, but verbal memory is typically impaired.

Anomic Aphasia (Semantic Dementia)

Just as right (greater than left) anterior temporal degeneration impairs the disambiguation of visually similar faces, left (greater than right) anterior temporal degeneration impairs lexical specification of an object—that is, the ability to name it. The term "semantic dementia" implies that with disease progression, the inability to name transcends the language domain and involves an actual loss of knowledge (17), but earlier in the course, the problem may reflect an inability to associate the still retrievable lexical tag with the intact concept of the object (18). In either case, patients have great difficulty naming specific objects. Figure 7.11 is an MRI of a patient's brain showing striking left (greater than right bilateral) anterior temporal atrophy. This pattern of atrophy is again more characteristic of a subtype of FTLD called semantic dementia (17) than of AD, but it can occur in either. Just as was noted for the right temporal variant (prosopagnosia), the difference largely reflects the age of the patient: semantic dementia in a 60-year-old most likely reflects FTLD but in an 80-year-old may reflect AD (16).

The problem is clinically more subtle than the grossly abnormal MRI might seem to imply. Patients are fluent, comprehend well, and can repeat, read, and write with minimal difficulty. Their speech lacks semantic precision, they substitute generic terms for specific words (e.g., "machine" for computer), and they make semantic paraphasias (e.g., "staple" for paperclip), but with passive listening, this type of naming deficit may go unnoticed. It is readily demonstrated, however, if the patient is actively confronted with specific common objects to name. (Neuropsychologists often use the Boston Naming Test, a series of 60 line drawings; such patients are typically very impaired on this test.) Although naming is characteristically impaired in most patients with typical AD, it is the disproportionate severity of impairment that distinguishes the anomic variant.

Mixed Aphasia

As the name implies, these patients have impairment of all aspects of language, making classification into a single taxonomic category impossible. Fluency, comprehension, naming, repetition, writing, and reading are all impaired. This pattern can appear early in a patient's course (Fig. 7.12), but more often emerges during the severe stage of dementia.

Asymmetrical Cortical Degeneration Syndromes: Apraxic Variants

In the setting of degenerative dementia, apraxia generally reflects parietal atrophy (Fig. 7.13).

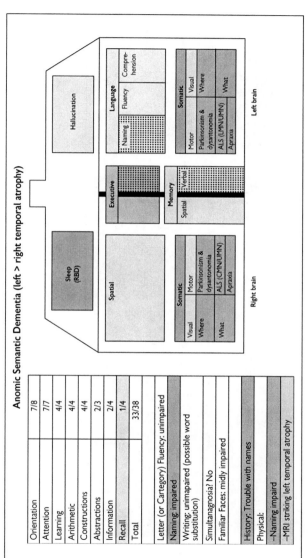

Anomic Semantic Dementia (left > right temporal atrophy)

Orientation	7/8
Attention	7/7
Learning	4/4
Arithmetic	4/4
Constructions	4/4
Abstractions	2/3
Information	2/4
Recall	1/4
Total	33/38

Letter (or Cartegory) Fluency: unimpaired

Naming: impaired

Writing: unimpaired (possible word substitution)

Simultanagnosia? No

Familiar Faces: midly impaired

History: Trouble with names

Physical:
- Naming: impaird
- MRI striking left temporal atrophy

Figure 7.11 Semantic dementia. Left anterior temporal lobe (and probably mild right as well) atrophy producing severe anomia and and verbal memory impairment in a 79 year old woman. Because neurodegeneration is usually bilateral, facial recognition may also become impaired with disease progression.

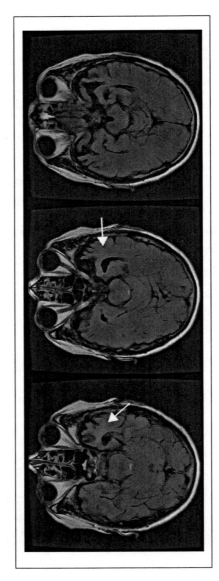

Figure 7.11 *Continued.*

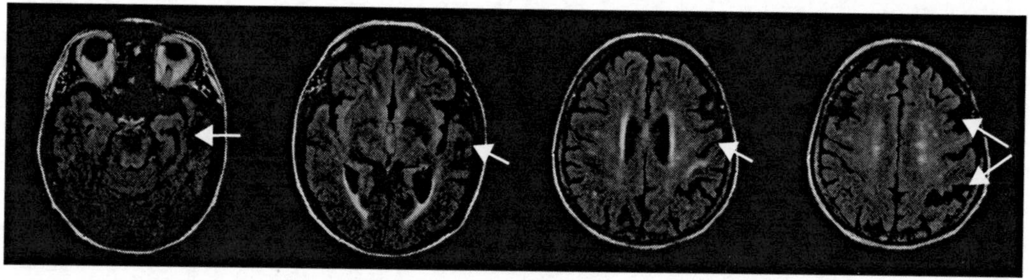

Figure 7.12 Mixed aphasia (aphasic variant Alzheimer's disease) with widespread asymmetric left hemispheric atrophy evident from inferior temporal to parietal vertex cortex in an 81 year old woman with a three year history of progressive memory loss and language difficulty.

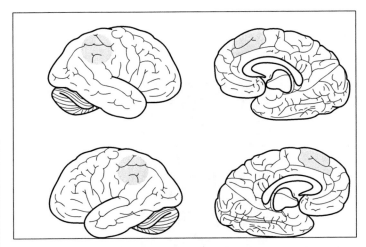

Figure 7.13 The syndrome of progressive apraxia reflects degeneration of parietal cortices and their connections, particularly to the supplemental motor area. Caselli RJ. Asymmetric cortical degeneration: syndromes and diseases. Neurologist 1995;1:1–20.

Of the major subtypes of apraxia, almost all cases occurring in the context of a degenerative dementia can be considered ideomotor (rather than ideational or motor), reflecting the impaired ability to translate intended goal-directed actions into functionally efficient movement. The types of functional tasks that are affected essentially define clinical severity. A patient whose sole impairment is impaired constructional skills has only mild disability, but a patient who can no longer dress himself or herself is severely impaired.

Figure 7.14 is an MRI of a patient's brain showing striking right (greater than left bilateral) parietal lobe atrophy.

This pattern of atrophy is most characteristic of corticobasal ganglionic degeneration (CBGD) but can also be produced by AD, progressive supranuclear palsy (PSP), and FTLD (19,20). All result in the syndrome of progressive apraxia, and it can be difficult to clinically distinguish the pathological subtypes. PSP often produces characteristic impairment of vertical eye movements (most often, patients cannot follow the examiner's finger up when eye movements are tested) that helps to distinguish it. CBGD itself produces not only apraxia that is quite asymmetrical, but often a severe hemiakinetic rigid syndrome that results eventually in a fixed dystonic-appearing clenched fist on the more severely affected side. AD, in contrast, is less asymmetrical, does not usually cause the hemirigidity of true CBGD, and causes more intellectual impairment (5). Patients retain insight into their impairment, however, and may appear less cognitively impaired than formal testing will reveal.

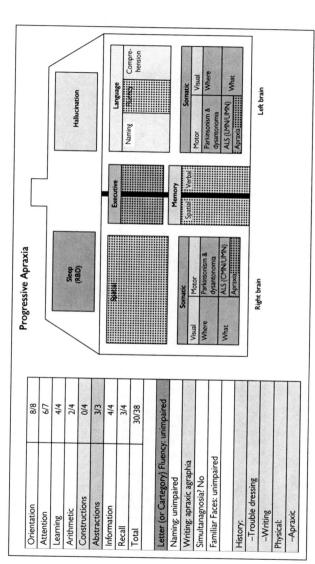

Figure 7.14 Apraxic variant Alzheimer's disease with right greater than left parietal atrophy evolving over 4 years in a 77 year old right handed woman. Apraxia is the most striking feature on neurological examination (gestural, dressing, constructional, and agraphic), but cognitive testing also often shows problems with executive skills and psychomotor speed.

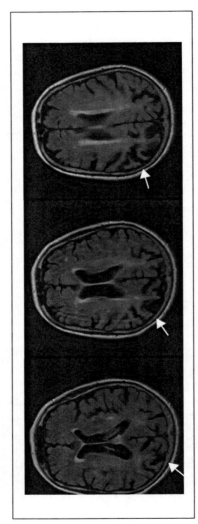

Figure 7.14 *Continued.*

To the extent that patients can move, they seem to no longer know how to perform a given movement, even though conceptually they seem to understand what is required and recall that they have previously been able to perform the task. Classical teaching defines apraxia as a disorder of skilled movement, and indeed, skilled movements such as using a fork and knife or a simple salute are impaired, but in the context of degenerative apraxia, even unskilled reaching and grasping (prehension) movements are impaired (5). More clinically relevant categories to evaluate include gestural apraxia (any movement involving limb gestures, such as pretending to brush one's teeth), dressing apraxia (such patients often will be dressed in clothes that can be pulled on to avoid buttons, laces, and clasps), constructional apraxia, and apraxic agraphia (Fig. 7.15). Patients are severely disabled by this disorder and require help with their activities of daily living beginning at a fairly early stage of their illness.

In addition to apraxia, other characteristic symptoms and signs may occur. Myoclonic jerks commonly occur, especially as the disease progresses to moderate and severe stages, but may be missing early on. Cortical sensory loss (tactile agnosia and astereognosis) occurs variably but sometimes can be quite severe, leading to the "alien limb" phenomenon in which the patient's limb will move seemingly of its own accord in a nondirected fashion when the patient is not aware.

The alien limb phenomenon is more common in patients with true CBGD than apraxic variant AD. Because the parietal lobes contain visually sensitive neurons in their posterior regions, some patients additionally develop asimultanagnosia (or a milder form of cortical visual impairment). When the more severely affected hemisphere is the language dominant (usually left) side, aphasia (and other left parietal deficits, such as acalculia) can result. Exceptionally, acalculia can even be an early presenting feature. Though highly inconsistent, it

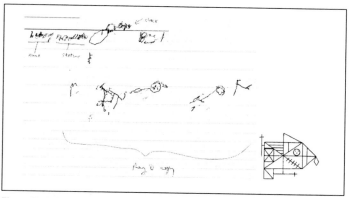

Figure 7.15 A 76 year old man with apraxic variant Alzheimer's disease with apraxic agraphia and constructional apraxia. Note at the top of the picture the patients attempt to write his name, a sentence, and draw a clock. In the bottom half of the Figure he has attempted to copy the Rey-Osterrieth Complex Figure pictured at the bottom right.

is strongly suggestive of a left inferior parietal focus when present (one such patient was a teacher who described an inability to grade her students' exams as a presenting feature of this syndrome). When instead the nondominant (usually right) hemisphere is more affected, there are greater spatial impairments. Hemispatial neglect can occur in this setting but is exceptional; when it does occur, a structural basis (e.g., superimposed cerebral infarction) should be excluded. Finally, most patients have significant psychomotor slowing that is evident on timed tests that ought not to be impaired by the motor deficit (e.g., the controlled oral word association test, or a category fluency test in which patients are asked to name as many animals as possible in a minute).

Asymmetrical Cortical Degeneration Syndromes: Dysexecutive Variants

This progressive neuropsychiatric syndrome is a characteristic subtype of FTLD that is associated with frontal and temporal lobe atrophy that is often asymmetrical (Fig. 7.16).

In the context of FTLD, the term for this syndrome is frontotemporal dementia. Pick's disease is prominently represented in the FTLD group, but the neuropathologically defining "Pick bodies" are an infrequent accompaniment, so that the more generic term FTLD is now used (21,22). As with the primary progressive nonfluent aphasia subtype, some FTLD patients with frontotemporal dementia develop motor neuron disease. AD is a less common cause of this syndrome, but again, the likelihood that such a patient will have underlying AD

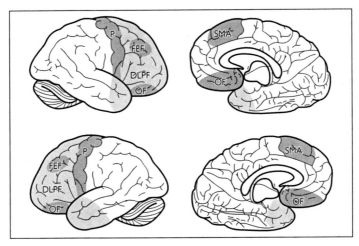

Figure 7.16 Dysexecutive syndromes reflect degeneration of anterior cortices including the frontal and anterior temporal lobes. Given the large size of these areas, and the diversity of functions encompassed, there is a similar range of disorders that may result from frontotemporal degeneration. Caselli RJ. Asymmetric cortical degeneration: syndromes and diseases. Neurologist 1995; 1:1–20.

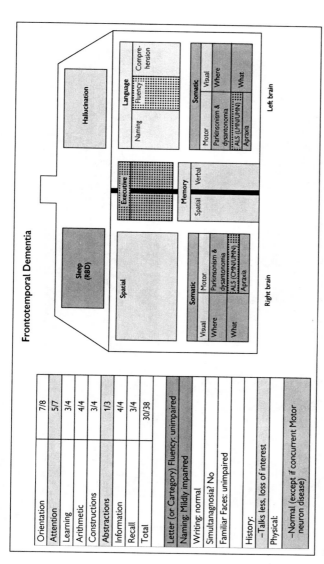

Figure 7.17 Progressive frontotemporal atrophy (right more than left) in a 76 year old man with a 3 year history of progressive apathy, inertia, mental slowing (with reduced letter fluency), and anomia. Memory loss is not prominent early on, but develops with disease progression. True FTLD patients develop motor neuron disease about 10% of the time, but patients with dysexecutive Alzheimer's disease do not.

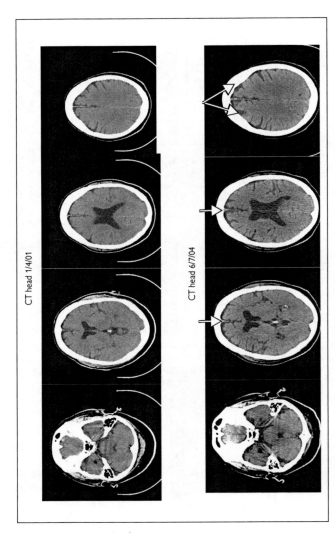

CT head 1/4/01

CT head 6/7/04

Figure 7.17 *Continued.*

depends on age: a 60-year-old will more likely have true FTLD, but an 80-year-old will more likely have a dysexecutive variant of AD (23,24) (Fig. 7.17).

Characteristic symptoms of the dysexecutive syndrome include abulia, a general reduction in interest and activity, so that patients talk less, walk more slowly, and seem less interested in reading or whatever may have been their previous interests. The errors of these patients tend to be omissions rather than commissions. They fail to change their clothes, brush their teeth, or initiate many of the activities that constitute a normal day. If prompted by someone else, however, they may be surprisingly capable of doing them, even when their initial response might be to say, "I can't" or "I don't know." Just as they fail to start something new, they may fail to stop what they are doing and perseveratively fixate, in a seemingly idiosyncratic fashion, on some particular activity, such as going to the bathroom, sorting through their wallet, or watching television. Some patients have greater disinhibition (Fig. 7.18) and emotional lability, crying or laughing at the least provocation.

Patients may complain they are hungry, yet be unmoved to fix themselves a snack. Some may perseveratively want to eat over and over, and coupled with their progressive inactivity, weight gain may occur, sometimes to a striking degree. Less often, patients may starve themselves from a lack of initiative to eat, although weight loss in the setting of a frontotemporal dementia syndrome should prompt a search for motor neuron disease and a swallowing study. Memory and language (especially naming) are typically impaired. There is often a reduced temporal latency in responding to the examiner. Patients may

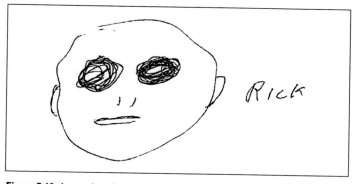

Figure 7.18 An unsolicited portrait of one of the authors by a disinhibited dementia patient spontaneously drawn during a followup visit.

even start answering a question before the physician has finished asking it, yet their answers are typically very terse.

References

1. Caselli RJ, Jack CR Jr. Asymmetric cortical degeneration syndromes: a proposed clinical classification. Arch Neurol 1992;49:770–780.

2. Caselli RJ, Jack CR Jr. Asymmetric cortical degeneration syndromes: clinical-radiological correlations. Neurology 1992;42:1462–1468.

3. Caselli RJ. Focal and asymmetric cortical degeneration syndromes. Adv Neurol 2000;82:35–51.

4. Caselli RJ. Asymmetric cortical degeneration syndromes. Curr Opin Neurol 1996;9:276–280.

5. Caselli RJ, Reiman EM, Timmann D, et al. Progressive apraxia in clinically discordant monozygotic twins. Arch Neurol 1995;52(10):1004–1010.

6. Caselli RJ. Visual syndromes as the presenting feature of degenerative brain disease. Sem Neurol 2000;20:139–144.

7. Tang-Wai DF, Graff-Radford RR, Boeve BF, et al. Clinical, genetic, and neuropathologic characteristics of posterior cortical atrophy. Neurology 2004;63:1168–1174.

8. McMonagle P, Deering F, Berliner Y, et al. The cognitive profile of posterior cortical atrophy. Neurology 2006;66:331–338.

9. Balint R. Seelenlahmung des "Schauens", optische Ataxie, raumliche Storung der Aufmerksamkeit. Monatssche Psychiat Neurol 1909;25:51–81.

10. Hodges JR. Frontotemporal dementia (Pick's disease): clinical features and assessment. Neurology 2001;56(11 Suppl 4):S6–10.

11. Snowden JS, Thompson JC, Neary D. Knowledge of famous faces and names in semantic dementia. Brain 2004;127(pt 4):860–872.

12. Joubert S, Felician O, Barbeau E, et al. Progressive prosopagnosia: clinical and neuroimaging results. Neurology 2004;63:1962–1965.

13. Pick A. On the relation between aphasia and senile atrophy of the brain. Translated by W.C. Schoene from: Pick A. Uber die Beziehungen der senilen Hirnatrophie zur Aphasie. Prager Medicinische Wochenschrift 17, 16 (1892), 165–167. In: Rottenberg DA, Hochberg FH, eds. Neurological Classics in Modern Translation. New York: Hafner Press, 1977:35–40.

14. Mesulam M. Primary progressive aphasia without generalized dementia. Ann Neurol 1982;11:592–598.

15. Josephs KA, Whitwell JL, Duffy JR, et al. Progressive aphasia secondary to Alzheimer disease vs FTLD pathology. Neurology 2008;70:25–34.

16. Knibb JA, Xuereb JH, Patterson K, et al. Clinical and pathological characterization of progressive aphasia. Ann Neurol 2006;59:156–165.

17. Hodges JR, Patterson K, Oxbury S, et al. Semantic dementia: progressive fluent aphasia with temporal lobe atrophy. Brain 1992;115(pt 6):1783–1806.

18. Caselli RJ, Ivnik RJ, Duffy JR. Associative anomia: dissociating words and their definitions. Mayo Clin Proc 1991;66(8):783–791.

19. Boeve BF, Maraganore DM, Parisi JE, et al. Pathologic heterogeneity in clinically diagnosed corticobasal degeneration. Neurology 1999;53:795–800.

20. Josephs KA, Tang-Wai DF, Edland SD, et al. Correlation between antemortem magnetic resonance imaging findings and pathologically confirmed corticobasal degeneration. Arch Neurol 2004;61:1881–1884.

21. Brun A. Frontal lobe degeneration of non-Alzheimer type. 1. Neuropathology. Arch Gerontol Geriatr 1987;6:193–208.

22. Gustafson L. Frontal lobe degeneration of non-Alzheimer type. II. Clinical picture and differential diagnosis. Arch Gerontol Geriatr 1987;6:209–223.

23. Alladi S, Xuereb J, Bak T, et al. Focal cortical presentations of Alzheimer's disease. Brain 2007;130(pt 10):2636–2645.

24. Snowden JS, Stopford CL, Julien CL, et al. Cognitive phenotypes in Alzheimer's disease and genetic risk. Cortex 2007;43:835–845.

Chapter 8

Neuropathological overlap syndromes

Association with Parkinson's Disease

Parkinson's disease and dementia overlap, and either can occur first. Among patients who initially develop parkinsonism, the prevalence of dementia increases with age and disease duration, so that among patients who have had Parkinson's disease for more than 20 years, 83% also have dementia (1). When cognitive decline begins at least a year after the onset of parkinsonism, by convention the diagnostic term used is "Parkinson's disease with dementia" (PDD). When instead cognitive decline begins within the first year of motor symptom onset, or when cognitive decline precedes the onset of parkinsonism, by convention the diagnostic term used is "dementia with Lewy bodies" (DLB) (2).

Neuropathologically there is little to no difference between PDD and DLB (3). Lewy bodies, intracytoplasmic inclusions composed of alpha-synuclein, are a defining feature of Parkinson's disease (4) (Fig. 8.1). In patients with Parkinson's disease, the Lewy bodies are concentrated in the brain stem catecholaminergic nuclei, principally the substantia nigra, locus ceruleus, and dorsal motor nucleus of the vagus nerve. In both PDD and DLB, Lewy bodies are found in these same regions but are also spread throughout the amygdala, entorhinal cortex,

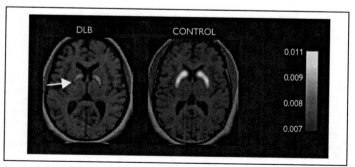

Figure 8.1 Reduced putamenal uptake of 6F-fluorodopa in a 59 year old woman with mild stage dementia with Lewy bodies.

and neocortex (2). In patients with either PDD or DLB, the characteristic neuropathological hallmarks of AD, neuritic plaques composed of abeta amyloid and neurofibrillary tangles, also occur in 50% to 75% of patients, far more than would be expected by chance alone (5–8). In fact the two are so closely associated that even among patients with neuropathologically confirmed clinical AD (and without parkinsonism), neocortical Lewy bodies can still be found in 25% to 60% of brains (9–12) (Fig. 8.2).

In both PDD and DLB, there is a characteristic tetrad of symptoms: parkinsonism, dementia, visual hallucinations, and REM sleep behavior disorder, a striking sleep disorder whose hallmark is dream enactment behavior (2) (Table 8.1).

The occurrence of visual hallucinations in patients with longstanding Parkinson's disease (with or without dementia) is often (but not always) a side effect of dopaminergic medications. However, the de novo onset of visual hallucinations in a seemingly healthy elder should prompt the diagnostic consideration of DLB. Symptoms of REM sleep behavior disorder can often be readily obtained by history if there is an available bed partner, but even in the absence of one, falling out of bed can be a clue (Fig. 8.3).

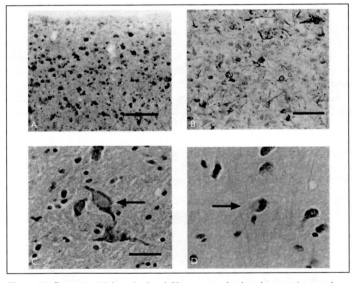

Figure 8.2 Dementia with Lewy bodies. A 58 yo woman developed progressive speech and language problems clinically diagnosed as primary progressive aphasia. At age 64 she developed paranoid delusions and visual hallucinations. At age 65 parkinsonism started. She died at age 69. Panels A and B show the signature pathologic features of Alzheimer's disease including amyloid plaques (A) and neurobigrillary tangles (B). Panels C and D show the signature features of synucleinopathies including Lewy bodies in the substantia nigra (C) and neocortex of the temporal lobe (D). Courtesy of Dr. Thomas Beach. From Caselli RJ, Beach TG, Sue LI, Connor DJ, Sabbagh MN. Progressive aphasia with Lewy bodies. Dement Geriatr Cogn Disord 2002; 14(2):55–8 (12). Reprinted with permission from S. Karger AG, Basel.

Table 8.1 Diagnostic Criteria for Dementia with Lewy Bodies

Central Feature

- Progressive cognitive decline that interferes with normal social and occupational function. Prominent or persistent memory impairment may not necessarily occur in the early stages but is usually evident with progression. Deficits on tests of attention, executive function, and visuospatial ability may be especially prominent.

Core Features (two for probable, one for possible DLB)

- Fluctuating cognition with pronounced variations in attention and alertness
- Recurrent visual hallucinations that are typically well formed and detailed
- Spontaneous features of parkinsonism

Suggestive Features (one or more in addition to one or more core features for probable, and in the absence of any core features for possible DLB)

- REM sleep behavior disorder (which may precede onset of dementia by several years)
- Severe neuroleptic sensitivity
- Abnormal (low uptake) in basal ganglia on SPECT or PET dopamine transporter scans

Supportive Features (commonly present but nonspecific)

- Repeated falls and syncope
- Transient, unexplained loss of consciousness
- Severe autonomic dysfunction (e.g., orthostatic hypotension, urinary incontinence)
- Hallucinations in other modalities
- Systematized delusions
- Depression
- Relative preservation of medial temporal lobe structures on CT/MRI scan
- Generalized low uptake on SPECT/PET perfusion scan with reduced occipital activity
- Abnormal (low uptake) MIBG myocardial scintigraphy
- Prominent slow wave activity on EEG with temporal lobe transient sharp waves

A diagnosis of DLB is less likely:

- In the presence of cerebrovascular disease evident as focal neurological signs or on brain imaging
- In the presence of any other physical illness or brain disorder sufficient to account in part or in total for the clinical picture
- If parkinsonism only appears for the first time at a stage of severe dementia

McKeith IG, Dickson DW, Loew J, et al. Diagnosis and management of dementia with Lewy bodies: third report of the DLB Consortium. Neurology 2005;65:1863–1872.

The characteristic cognitive profile of dementia in patients with parkinsonism includes impaired learning and memory, psychomotor slowing, constructional apraxia, and more profound visual spatial impairment than in similarly staged AD patients (13). When treating hallucinations in such patients (see the section on pharmacotherapy), it is important to realize that patients with DLB may have greater extrapyramidal sensitivity to antipsychotic medications than those with pure AD (2). While all patients with dementia experience day-to-day fluctuations in symptom severity, such fluctuations can be more exaggerated in DLB patients.

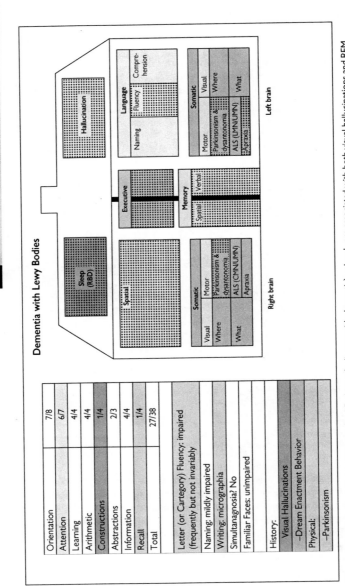

Figure 8.3 Dementia with Lewy bodies (and Parkinson's disease with dementia) uniquely are associated with both visual hallucinations and REM Sleep Behavior Disorder as well as parkinsonism and a pattern of dementia with mixed cortical and subcortical (psychomotor slowing) features.

Association with Vascular Dementia

The terminology for cognitive impairment occurring within the setting of cerebrovascular disease has been almost as confusing as the disease itself. Proposed diagnostic criteria for vascular dementia mandate the presence of dementia with clinical and radiological stroke-like features that include focal signs and visualized infarctions. The cognitive manifestations of vascular dementia include psychomotor slowing and executive dysfunction, while somatic manifestations include gait impairment that resembles parkinsonism (14–16). Vascular mechanisms of cognitive loss include the direct consequences of brain infarctions, hemorrhages, and global hypoxia–ischemia. Since at least the days of Broca and Wernicke, it has been clear that cerebral infarction can impair cognitive skills, and prior to the current age of functional neuroimaging, cognitive neuroscientists frequently used the "lesion method" to study brain–behavior relationships (Fig. 8.4).

Among patients with cognitive decline, vascular pathology is common and often coexists with AD. Realizing the importance of cognitive decline as an outcome shared by multiple disease mechanisms, Hachinski proposed the concept of vascular cognitive impairment that ranges from a brain "at risk" due to atherosclerotic risk factors and small vessel-type abnormalities on neuroimaging studies ("leukoaraiosis") to the most extreme form of multiple large artery territory infarctions (17,18). This has fostered a collaboration between cognitive and vascular neurologists that emphasizes the overlap of risk factors and outcomes of AD and cerebrovascular disease (19). Respecting the spectrum of vascular diseases that may result in cognitive impairment, we will consider three main forms of "vascular cognitive impairment," two of which in particular have a special relationship to AD.

Small Vessel Atherosclerotic Vascular Dementia

Vascular dementia has historically referred to a disorder less obvious than one as diagnostically straightforward as a single stroke, one that reflects impaired blood and oxygen delivery in a multifocal or diffuse fashion at the microvascular level of cerebral circulation. In most cases, this is associated with well-recognized cerebrovascular risk factors that include hypertension, diabetes mellitus, hypercholesterolemia, tobacco smoking, and a family history of stroke. Treatment of these factors has reduced the incidence of cerebral infarction, and therefore it is hoped may slow the progression of small vessel atherosclerotic vascular dementia. While some patients do report an abrupt stroke-like event, many patients with this form of vascular dementia instead report steadily progressive decline (20). The clinical pattern has a somewhat "subcortical" appearance with slowed cognition and movement (resembling very mild parkinsonism but without the rest tremor), impaired learning and recall, and relative preservation of language (20,21). Patients may appear depressed, although in some this may simply reflect psychomotor slowing. Radiologically, these patients often (but not invariably) have extensive subcortical white and gray matter lesions (termed

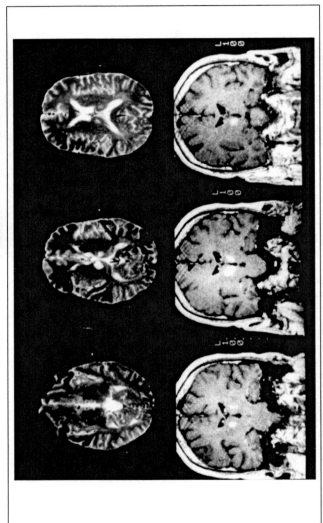

Figure 8.4 Bilateral thalamic infarctions causing amnesia in a 66 year old man. This is one example of how cerebral infarctions can impair cognition, sometimes in a pattern that might be mistaken for Alzheimer's disease.

Reprinted from Caselli RJ, Graff-Radford NR, Rezai K. Thalamocortical diaschisis: a single photon emission tomography (SPET) study of cortical perfusion changes following focal thalamic infarctions. Neuropsychiatry Neuropsychol Behav Neurol 1991; 4:193–214.

leukoaraiosis on CT and a variety of terms such as small vessel disease or multiple lacunar infarcts on MRI (Fig. 8.5).

Neuropathologically, some lesions are indeed small lacunar infarctions, but more are ischemic areas characterized by neuronal loss, demyelination, and gliosis without the frank cavitation of a lacunar infarction (22). In addition, the majority have concurrent AD (23–25).

Single or Multiple Large Artery Territory Infarctions with Vascular Cognitive Impairment

In this large artery type, clinically evident strokes occur with consequent accrual of deficits. This is not a slowly progressive disease but one of defined events. An ongoing controversy, however, is whether AD develops at an accelerated rate following (and by implication as a result of) cerebral infarction (or hemorrhage) (26,27). Recent investigations have also suggested that risk factors for atherosclerotic vascular disease are risk factors for AD, and that there is also a statistically significant association with atherosclerosis of major intracranial arteries (28,29). To date, however, the results of epidemiological studies are mixed. The incidence and prevalence of dementia is higher following cerebral infarction, but this appears to be due primarily to vascular pathology and not AD (30,31).

Amyloid Angiopathy

Just as amyloid may abnormally deposit in brain parenchyma, so too may it deposit in the walls of penetrating cerebral and dural arteries. In doing so it causes abnormal permeability of the blood–brain barrier, a reduced caliber of the arterial lumen, and a weakening of the arterial media. This leads to similar ischemic changes as its atherosclerotic small vessel counterpart, but additionally predisposes to massive and sometimes recurrent lobar intracerebral hemorrhages. Such hemorrhages tend to be located in the posterior hemispheres, in areas that would be uncharacteristic for hypertensive intracerebral hemorrhage. Even in the absence of such lobar hemorrhages, MRI-based diffusion-weighted images reveal multiple punctate areas of "microhemorrhage" or hemosiderin deposition, yielding a diagnostically characteristic pattern (Fig. 8.6).

Amyloid angiopathy can occur as a separate entity, but when present in a patient with cognitive impairment suggests the coexistence of AD (32–35). There is, unfortunately, no known treatment to reduce the progression of amyloid angiopathy, and because such patients are already at elevated risk for lobar hemorrhages, anticoagulant (36) (and possibly antiplatelet [37]) therapy may further escalate the risk. Rarely patients with AD may present with a focal syndrome and an MRI appearance suggesting a mass lesion (Fig. 8.7). While a true brain tumor should always be considered first, some patients neuropathologically have been found to have excessive amyloid deposition in brain parenchyma, amyloid angiopathy with perivascular lymphocytic inflammation (which may include multinucleated giant cells), and local cerebral edema (38).

Finally, other causes of cerebrovascular disease may also lead to cognitive impairment in the absence of any association with AD. These include

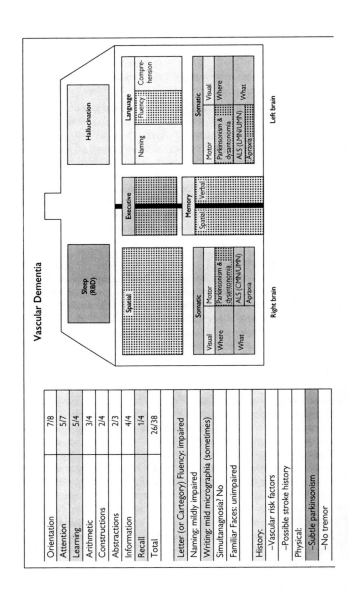

Orientation	7/8
Attention	5/7
Learning	5/4
Arithmetic	3/4
Constructions	2/4
Abstractions	2/3
Information	4/4
Recall	1/4
Total	26/38

Letter (or Cartegory) Fluency: impaired

Naming: mildly impaired

Writing: mild micrographia (sometimes)

Simultanagnosia? No

Familiar Faces: unimpaired

History:
– Vascular risk factors
– Possible stroke history

Physical:
– Subtle parkinsonism
– No tremor

Vascular Dementia

Sleep (RBD)

Hallucination

Spatial

Executive

Language

Naming | Fluency | Compre-hension

Memory

Spatial | Verbal

Somatic

Visual | Motor | Parkinsonism & dysantonomia

Where | ALS (CMN/UMN)

What | Apraxia

Somatic

Motor | Visual

Parkinsonism & dysantonomia | Where

ALS (LMN/UMN) | What

Apraxia

Right brain

Left brain

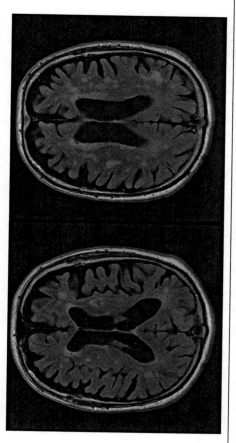

Figure 8.5 Small vessel atherosclerotic vascular dementia in an 83 year old hypertensive, hyperlipidemic man with mild stage dementia. Vascular dementia is characterized by impaired executive skills, psychomotor speed, learning (and recall to a lesser degree) with physical features resembling mild parkinsonism.

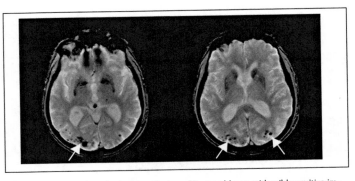

Figure 8.6 Cerebral amyloid angiopathy in an 82 year old man with mild cognitive impairment. The black spots on this diffusion weighted MRI are focal hemosiderin deposits. Their posterior predominance reflects the tendency for intracerebral |hemorrhages to occur in posterior cerebral regions, unlike typical and more common hypertensive intracerebral hemorrhages.

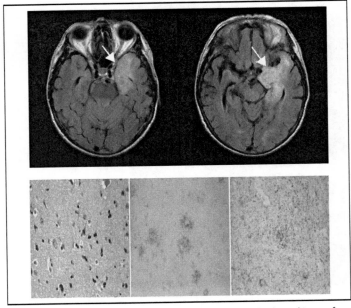

Figure 8.7 "Amyloidoma". A 75 year old woman presented with a 5 year history of slowly progressive memory decline (first evaluated in 1997), and a 2 year history of personality change and mild word finding difficulty. MRI in 1997 was normal, but in 2002 (pictured above) showed an infiltrative appearing lesion in the left temporal lobe. Biopsy is shown beneath the MRI including, from left to right, H&E, antibody to amyloid, and tau stains that are consistent with Alzheimer's disease (courtesy of Dr. Dennis Dickson). There was no evidence of a tumor.

hematological disorders that lead to a hypercoagulable state, cerebral auto-somal dominant arteriopathy with subcortical infarcts and leukoencephalopa-thy (CADASIL), and cerebral (both primary and secondary) vasculitis.

References

1. Hely MA, Reid WG, Adena MA, et al. The Sydney multicenter study of Parkinson's disease: the inevitability of dementia at 20 years. Mov Disord 2008;23:837–844.

2. McKeith IG, Dickson DW, Loew J, et al. Diagnosis and management of dementia with Lewy bodies: third report of the DLB Consortium. Neurology 2005;65:1863–1872.

3. Lippa CF, Duda JE, Grossman M, et al. DLB and PDD boundary issues: diagnosis, treatment, molecular pathology, and biomarkers. Neurology 2007;68:812–819.

4. Goedert M. Alpha-synuclein and neurodegerative diseases. Nat Rev Neurosci 2001;2:492–501.

5. Verghese J, Crystal HA, Dickson DW, et al. Validity of clinical criteria for the diagnosis of dementia with Lewy bodies. Neurology 1999;53:1974–1982.

6. Hohl U, Tiraboschi P, Hansen LA, et al. Diagnostic accuracy of dementia with Lewy bodies. Arch Neurol 2000;57:347t–351.

7. Dickson DW. Dementia with Lewy bodies: neuropathology. J Geriatr Psychiatry Neurol 2002;15:210–216.

8. Iseki E. Dementia with Lewy bodies: reclassification of pathological subtypes and boundary with Parkinson's disease or Alzheimer's disease. Neuropathology 2004;24:72–78.

9. Kotzbauer PT, Trojanowsk JQ, Lee VM. Lewy body pathology in Alzheimer's disease. J Mol Neurosci 2001;17:225–232.

10. Gomez-Tortosa E, Ingraham AO, Irizarry MC, et al. Dementia with Lewy bodies. J Am Geriatr Soc 1998;46:1449–1458.

11. Joachim CL, Morris JH, Selkoe DJ. Clinically diagnosed Alzheimer's disease. Autopsy results in 150 cases. Ann Neurol 1988;24:50–56.

12. Caselli RJ, Beach TG, Sue LI, et al. Progressive aphasia with Lewy bodies. Dement Geriatr Cogn Disord 2002;14(2):55–58. 13. Ferman TJ, Boeve BF, Smith GE, et al. REM sleep behavior disorder and dementia: cognitive differences when compared with AD. Neurology 1999;52:951–957.

14. Roman GC, Tatemichi TK, Erkinjuntti T, et al. Vascular dementia: diagnostic criteria for research studies. Report of the NINDS-AIREN international workshop. Neurology 1993;43:250–260.

15. Chui HC, Victoroff JI, Margolin D, et al. Criteria for the diagnosis of ischemic vascular dementia proposed by the State of California Alzheimer's Disease Diagnostic and Treatment Centers. Neurology 1992;42:473–480.

16. Chui HC, Mack W, Jackson JE, et al. Clinical criteria for the diagnosis of vascular dementia: a multicenter study of comparability and interrater reliability. Arch Neurol 2000;57:191–196.

17. Hachinski V. Vascular dementia: a radical redefinition. Dementia 1994;5:130–132.

18. Hachinski V. The 2005 Thomas Willis Lecture: stroke and vascular cognitive impairment: a transdisciplinary, translational, and transactional approach. Stroke 2007;38:1396–1403.

19. Hachniski V, Iadecola C, Petersen RC, et al. National Institute of Neurological Disorders and Stroke-Canadian Stroke Network Vascular Cognitive Impairment Harmonization Standards. Stroke 2006;37:2220–2241.

20. Reed BR, Mungas DM, Kramer JH, et al. Clinical and neuropsychological features in autopsy-defined vascular dementia. Clin Neuropsychol 2004;18:63–74.

21. Chui HC. Subcortical ischemic vascular dementia. Neurol Clin 2007;25:717–740.

22. Young VG, Halliday GM, Kril JJ. Neuropathologic correlates of white matter hyperintensities. Neurology 2008;71:804–811.

23. Korczyn AD. Mixed dementia: the most common form of dementia. Ann NY Acad Sci 2002;977:129–134.

24. Nolan KA, Lino MM, Seligmann AW, et al. Absence of vascular dementia in an autopsy series from a dementia clinic. J Am Geriatr Soc 1998;46:597–604.

25. Hulette C, Nochlin D, McKeel D, et al. Clinical-neuropathologic findings in multi-infarct dementia: a report of six autopsied cases. Neurology 1997;48:668–672.

26. Honig LS, Tang MX, Albert S, et al. Stroke and the risk of Alzheimer disease. Arch Neurol 2003;60:1707–1712.

27. Schneider JA, Wilson RS, Bienias JL, et al. Cerebral infarctions and the likelihood of dementia from Alzheimer disease pathology. Neurology 2004;62:1148–1155.

28. Roher AE, Esh C, Rahman A, et al. Atherosclerosis of cerebral arteries in Alzheimer disease. Stroke 2004;35:2623–2627.

29. Honig LS, Kukull W, Mayeux R. Atherosclerosis and AD: analysis of data from the US National Alzheimer's Coordinating Center. Neurology 2005;64:494–500.

30. Hayden KM, Zandi PP, Lyketsos CG, et al. Vascular risk factors for incident Alzheimer disease and vascular dementia: the Cache County study. Alzheimer Dis Assoc Disord 2006;20:93–100.

31. Schneider JA, Boyle PA, Arvanitakis Z, et al. Subcortical infarcts, Alzheimer's disease pathology, and memory function in older persons. Ann Neurol 2007;62:59–66.

32. Haglund M, Sjobeck M, Englund E. Severe amyloid angiopathy characterizes an underestimated variant of vascular dementia. Dementia Geriatr Cogn Disord 2004;18:132–137.

33. Thal DR, Ghebremedhin E, Orantes M, et al. Vascular pathology in Alzheimer disease: correlation of cerebral amyloid angiopathy and arteriosclerosis/lipohyalinosis with cognitive decline. J Neuropathol Exp Neurol 2003;62:1287–1301.

34. Tian J, Shi J, Bailey K, et al. Association between apolipoprotein E e4 allele and arteriosclerosis, cerebral amyloid angiopathy, and cerebral white matter damage in Alzheimer's disease. J Neurol Neurosurg Psychiatry 2004;75:696–699.

35. Nicoll JA, Yamada M, Frackowiac J, et al. Cerebral amyloid angiopathy plays a direct role in the pathogenesis of Alzheimer's disease. Pro-CAA position statement. Neurobiol Aging 2004;25:589–597.

36. Lee SH, Ryu WS, Roh JK. Cerebral microbleeds are a risk factor for warfarin-related intracerebral hemorrhage. Neurology 2009;72:171–176.

37. Wong KS, Chan YL, Liu JY, et al. Asymptomatic microbleeds as a risk factor for aspirin-associated intracerebral hemorrhages. Neurology 2003;60:511–513.

38. Eng JA, Frosch MP, Choi K, et al. Clinical manifestations of cerebral amyloid angiopathy-related inflammation. Ann Neurol 2004;55:250–256.

Pharmacotherapy of Alzheimer's disease (and other forms of dementia): a practical approach to medical management

At the time of this writing, AD cannot be cured. However, because it is a progressive disease, evolving from its mildest to most severe stages over the course of years, patients diagnosed at an early stage still have a lot of living left to do. The general principles of management are to slow and smooth the expected progression of symptoms and disability, mitigate foreseeable risks, maximize the patient's quality of life, and most importantly help the family (and/or others) to succeed in their role as primary caregivers. Treatment success (and failure) ultimately depends more of the quality of the patient's support from family, friends, and professional caregivers than from the cleverness and good intentions of their physicians.

Medications that have FDA approval for the specific treatment of AD are those that address the cognitive disorder and are discussed in Chapter 9. Behavioral problems, another major source of symptomatic impairment, are discussed in Chapter 10, with the explicit advisory that the medications discussed are off-label for AD. Finally, a variety of other issues, including sleep disturbances, common comorbidities, abrupt decline, and prevention, are discussed in Chapter 11. (Nonpharmacotherapeutic interventions are discussed in Section D.)

In summary, there are six pharmacotherapeutic categories of concern to be addressed in patients with dementia, although not each category will require intervention in every patient:

1. Intellectual decline
2. Behavioral disorders
3. Sleep disorders
4. Comorbid conditions
5. Abrupt decline
6. Prevention (primary and secondary)

Table C.1 provides a basic clinical guide to the types of management issues clinicians should address with each patient at each visit, because these issues influence management decisions and the quality of life for both patient and caregiver.

Table C.1 Pharmacotherapy of Alzheimer's Disease: Outline

	FDA Approved	Other/Off-Label
Intellectual Decline		
Mild/moderate stage	Donepezil	
	Rivastigmine	Patch available
	Galantamine	Generic available
Moderate/severe stage	Memantine	
	Donepezil	
Behavioral Problems		
Depression	SSRIs preferred	
Anxiety	SSRIs, buspirone	Antipsychotics
Agitation, aggression, and psychosis	None	Antipsychotics
Sleep Disorders		
Insomnia	Zolpidem, zaleplon, etc.	Trazodone
REM behavior disorder	None	Clonazepam
Obstructive sleep apnea	CPAP	
Nocturia	Oxybutynin, tolterodine	Intermittent catheterization
Common Comorbidities		
Parkinsonism	Levodopa/carbidopa, etc.	Rx only if necessary
Incontinence	Oxybutynin, tolterodine	Intermittent catheterization
Dysphagia	None	Advance directives
Abrupt Decline		
Community	Evaluate	Infections, medication errors, etc.
Hospital/postoperative	Evaluate	Antipsychotics, etc.
Prevention		
	None	Physical fitness, manage comorbidities, Mediterranean diet, etc.

Chapter 9

Pharmacotherapy: cognitive impairment

Dementia therapy has had a rocky road. Cognitive impairment such as memory loss represents the only target of FDA-approved pharmacotherapy and is reviewed here. Behavioral disorders and their management will be considered separately. Even today, the noncognitive manifestations of AD are not accepted by the FDA as legitimate primary therapeutic targets for demonstrating efficacy, leaving many patients, families, and clinicians to struggle with less standardized approaches. Prior to the 1970s, clinical experience and prevailing theories of aging and dementia led to the use of psychostimulants, vasodilators, ergoloids, and various combinations of drugs. In the United States, dihydroergotoxin mesylate, a putative cerebral vasodilator, was approved by the FDA for "senile mental decline," and its use was prevalent through the 1980s until controlled trials demonstrated its inefficacy. The development in the 1980s of standardized research-based diagnostic criteria for AD (1), coupled with initial insights into its pathophysiology, led to the development of mechanism-based pharmacotherapeutics and randomized, controlled clinical trials that ushered in the first clinically proven effective therapies (Table 9.1).

Not all medications are equally effective for stages of dementia severity, and FDA approvals for individual agents reflect this. Two of the four in widespread use are approved for severe dementia, and three for mild-stage dementia. Disease severity can be determined with a variety of research tools, but in clinical practice, the mental status examination and activities of daily living are relied upon most often. The following two vignettes illustrate the two ends of the severity spectrum; this will allow us to consider which medications are appropriate in which setting.

Vignette A: Mild- to Moderate-Stage Dementia

An 84-year-old woman has mild-stage Alzheimer's dementia. Her MMSE score is 22/30. She repeats herself, has trouble recalling the names of familiar people, and usually forgets where she placed her glasses. She has no difficulties with dressing or bathing. She still cooks, although her meals are less complex than they have been in the past, and she cannot work the microwave. Her family is wondering if there is anything that might improve her memory so that she does

Table 9.1 FDA-Approved Drugs for the Treatment of Alzheimer's Disease

Drug	Indication	How Supplied	Initial Dosage	Maintenance Dosage	Comments
Donepezil	Mild to severe AD	5- and 10-mg tablets and orally dispersable tablets	5 mg daily	5–10 mg daily	5 and 10 mg/day are both effective doses, 10 mg possibly slightly more so
Rivastigmine	Mild to moderate AD	1.5-, 3-, 4.5-, and 6-mg capsules; transdermal patch 4.6 and 9.5 mg	Capsules 1.5 mg bid; patch 4.6 mg daily	Capsules 3, 4.5, or 6 mg bid; patch 9.5 mg daily	Take with food. Effective dose range: oral 3–6 mg bid or 9.5 mg patch.
Galantamine	Mild to moderate AD	4-, 8-, and 12-mg tablets; solution 4 mg/mL; 8-, 12-, and 24-mg extended-release capsules	4 mg bid; extended-release 8 mg daily	8 or 12 mg bid; extended-release 16 or 24 mg daily	Generic available. Effective dose range: 16–24 mg daily.
Memantine	Moderate to Severe AD	5- and 10-mg capsules	5 mg daily (4 week titration pack)	10 mg bid	NMDA receptor antagonist

not repeat herself quite so much, can recall her grandchildren's names, can find her glasses, and maybe can even learn to use the microwave.

Vignette B: Moderate- to Severe-Stage Dementia

An 86-year-old man has moderately severe dementia caused by AD. His MMSE score is 11/30. He has difficulty expressing himself, and his comprehension seems inconsistent. In addition, over the past 6 months he has needed assistance dressing himself. He still can feed himself and bathe, although both activities are taking longer and he now makes occasional mistakes such as using a spoon instead of a knife, and not washing as thoroughly as he should. His family is wondering if it might be possible to restore or preserve his level of function so that he might continue to perform his basic activities of daily living himself without requiring assistance from others.

The Acetylcholinesterase Inhibitors

Neurotransmitter perturbations provide accessible targets for therapeutic interventions. In AD patients, cerebral choline acetyltransferase (ChAT) activity, the key enzyme in acetylcholine (Ach) synthesis (2–4), is reduced, and there is a loss of cholinergic neurons in the basal forebrain that includes the nucleus basalis of Meynert (5,6), both of which contribute to a neurotransmitter deficiency of Ach. The degree of loss of cortical ChAT activity and nucleus basalis neurons correlates pathologically with neocortical amyloid plaque density (7,8), and clinically with dementia severity (9). Among patients whose clinical course is complicated by depression, another neuronal system that is affected is the nucleus locus ceruleus (nLC), which releases serotonin (10,11), particularly in AD patients whose course is complicated by depression (12,13). Similarly, demented patients with major depression also have a tenfold reduction in norepinephrine compared to their nondepressed counterparts (14). (Depression, however, is not a primary target for dementia therapy.)

Ach is inactivated when it is hydrolyzed to choline and acetate by acetylcholinesterase (AChE). Acetylcholinesterase inhibitors (AChEIs) effectively increase the amount of ACh available for intrasynaptic cholinergic receptor stimulation. Butyrylcholinesterase (BuChE) also hydrolyzes ACh. AChE projections are thought to modulate cortical processing and responses to new stimuli; BuCHE-positive neurons project principally to the frontal cortex, perhaps influencing attention, executive function, emotional memory, and behavior (15). An AChEI can work at either of two sites on AChE: an ionic subsite or a catalytic esteratic subsite to prevent the interaction between ACh and AChE. Early clinical trials of physostigmine, an AChEI, produced modest improvement in memory (16–19), but its utility was limited by adverse reactions and frequent dosing. Early success with dosage individualization (20) led to multicenter trials of the AChEIs tacrine, velnacrine, and sustained-release physostigmine (21–23) and subsequently provided the rationale and justification for larger clinical trials and eventual FDA approval of tacrine (although with the advent of newer agents, tacrine is no longer actively marketed due to its difficult dosing regimen, poor tolerability, and significant hepatotoxicity) (24). The newer AChEIs donepezil, rivastigmine, and galantamine are a mainstay of current dementia therapy.

Tacrine and donepezil act at the ionic subsite. Rivastigmine acts at the catalytic esteratic subsite (25). Galantamine acts at both the ionic site and catalytic binding site (15). Donepezil and galantamine are relatively selective for AChE (26), whereas tacrine and rivastigmine inhibit both AChE and BuChE. Binding to the AChE sites may be either reversible or irreversible, and may be competitive or noncompetitive with acetylcholine. Galantamine is an example of a competitive AChEI, competing with acetylcholine for AChE. In addition, AChE is present in a few molecular forms containing one (monomeric G1), two (dimeric G2), or four (tetrameric G4) catalytic subunits. The G1 and G4 forms are present in varying proportion in different brain regions (27). The tetrameric G4 is located on the presynaptic membranes within the cholinergic synaptic cleft; the monomeric G1 is found on postsynaptic membranes. While G4 is decreased with the loss of presynaptic cholinergic neurons, postsynaptic cholinergic receptor neurons and G1 Ach are not decreased significantly with AD or aging (25). Similar to AChE, BuChE exists in G1, G2, and G4 molecular forms, with a preponderance of the G4 isoform in the brain (28). The BuChE monomeric G1 increases by 30% to 60% in the Alzheimer brain, whereas the BuChE tetrameric G4 isoform decreases or remains the same. Thus, investigations of AChEI should consider the molecular form-specific characteristics of AChE and BuChE inhibition. Rivastigmine is an AChEI that is highly selective for the postsynaptic G1 monomer form of AChE, while galantamine is less so, and donepezil is not.

Donepezil

Donepezil is a long-acting piperidine-based highly selective and reversible AChEI. Two phase III clinical trials (29,30) resulted in FDA approval for early to moderate stages of AD in late 1996. Subsequent randomized clinical trials have included a trial of 6 months' duration (31), a Scandinavian study of 12 months (32), a study of nursing home patients (33), a trial assessing functional decline (34), and a 6-month trial in which a large proportion of patients were more severely impaired than in previous trials (35). Two 24-week clinical trials conducted in nursing home patients in Sweden (36) and outpatients in Japan (37) with severe AD provided sufficient cognitive and global efficacy for the FDA to approve donepezil for this indication in 2006. Donepezil is currently the only AChEI with FDA approval for the treatment of severe AD. A trial sponsored by the UK's Medical Research Council confirmed the modest benefits in cognition and activities of daily life over a 2-year period with a modal donepezil dose of 5 mg/day. However, it did not demonstrate that donepezil delayed time to nursing home placement or progression of disability (38). Despite methodological limitations, the trial results undermined assumptions that such improvements in cognition and daily activities translated to cost effectiveness of treatment or a meaningful delay in institutionalization. Donepezil may decrease the rate of hippocampal atrophy in AD (39), although this was not found in patients with mild cognitive impairment (40).

Donepezil is initiated at 5 mg daily and then increased to 10 mg daily after 4 to 6 weeks. The most common gastrointestinal side effects of donepezil include nausea, vomiting, diarrhea, and anorexia. Some patients develop muscle cramps, headache, dizziness, syncope, flushing, insomnia, weakness, drowsiness, fatigue, and agitation. Weight loss of more than 7% of baseline occurred at twice the rate of placebo in the nursing home study, but not in outpatient trials. Adverse effects occur at higher rates when the titration from 5 to 10 mg was made in 1 week compared to 6 weeks. When taken at bedtime, vivid dreams and nightmares may occur that can be relieved in most instances with morning dosing instead of bedtime.

Rivastigmine

Rivastigmine is a pseudo-irreversible, selective AChE subtype inhibitor. Although it inhibits butyrylcholinesterase as well, it is relatively selective for the postsynaptic G1 monomer form of AChE in areas of the neocortex and hippocampus. After binding to AChE, the carbamate portion of rivastigmine is slowly hydrolyzed, cleaved, conjugated to a sulfate, and excreted. Thus, its metabolism is essentially extrahepatic and is unlikely to have significant pharmacokinetic interactions. Four phase III randomized, placebo-controlled, 26-week-long clinical trials were completed of similar design, but differing mainly in dosing methods. Two have been published (41,42). Some results of the third trial have been included in secondary reports (43–46). In the two published trials, doses were titrated weekly during the first 7 weeks to one of two dosage ranges, 1 to 4 mg/day or 6 to 12 mg/day, and dose decreases were not permitted, possibly contributing to lesser tolerability during these stages of treatment. A 6-month, multicenter trial of transdermal rivastigmine showed that the patch provided similar benefits to oral rivastigmine. At lower doses transdermal administration was better tolerated than oral administration, but not at higher doses (47).

The recommended starting dose of rivastigmine is 1.5 mg twice daily, taken with meals, increasing to 3 mg twice daily after a minimum of 2 weeks of treatment and only if the initial dose is well tolerated. Subsequent increases to 4.5 mg and then 6 mg twice daily are based on good tolerability with the previous dose and may be considered after a minimum 2-week treatment interval. Rivastigmine is also available as an oral solution and a transdermal patch. Transdermal rivastigmine is started with an initial 4.6-mg patch per day for at least 4 weeks before the dose is raised to a 9.5-mg patch per day, again based on good tolerability with the previous dose. Adverse effects are primarily gastrointestinal and led to withdrawal in one study in 23% of the high-dose group (6 to 12 mg total daily dose), 7% of the low-dose group, and 7% of the placebo group. Other adverse effects in the higher-dose group during dose escalation were sweating, fatigue, asthenia, weight loss, malaise, dizziness, somnolence, nausea, vomiting, anorexia, and flatulence. In the maintenance phase, dizziness, nausea, vomiting, dyspepsia, and sinusitis occurred more in the high-dose group than in the placebo group. The FDA approval letter requested that the manufacturer do further analyses to better characterize these effects, especially weight loss and anorexia.

Galantamine

Galantamine, an alkaloid originally extracted from Amaryllidaceae (*Galanthus woronowi*, the Caucasian snowdrop) but now synthesized, is a reversible, competitive inhibitor of AChE with relatively little butyrylcholinesterase activity (48). Competitive inhibitors compete with Ach at AChE binding sites, so their inhibition is, theoretically, dependent on intrasynaptic ACh. Another characteristic is its allosteric modulation of nicotinic receptor sites, thus possibly enhancing cholinergic transmission by presynaptic nicotinic stimulation (49). Four multicenter trials, involving over 2,400 subjects (50–53), and a systematic review (54) have been published. The results of two trials indicated that treatment with either 24 or 32 mg/day of galantamine improved cognition, the clinician's global assessment of change, and ADL scores, with fewer adverse effects at the lower dose. The results of the third trial showed that daily doses of 16 mg or 24 mg were effective, but the 8-mg dosage was not.

Initial dosing of the original formulation of galantamine is 4 mg twice daily; this should be raised to 8 mg twice daily after 2 to 4 weeks. For patients who are tolerating medication but not responding, the dose can be raised to 12 mg twice daily after another 4 weeks. The FDA approved galantamine in April 2001 under the trade name Reminyl. Due to confusion with the diabetes medication glimepiride (Amaryl), in 2005 the trade name Reminyl was changed to Razadyne. An extended-release formulation of galantamine (Razadyne ER) was subsequently FDA approved for once-daily use (55). The extended-release formulation of galantamine is started at 8 mg/day, and the dosage is increased to 16 mg/day after 4 weeks. After 4 weeks, the dosage can be further increased to 24 mg/day based upon clinical benefit and tolerability. The Cochrane Database of Systematic Reviews found that 16 mg/day showed statistically indistinguishable efficacy from higher doses (54). Principal adverse effects are nausea, vomiting, diarrhea, anorexia, weight loss, abdominal pain, dizziness, and tremor. Again, adverse events were more common earlier in the course of treatment and during the dosage titration from 16 to 24 mg/day and higher. In one trial the effective dosage of 16 mg/day was not associated with overall greater adverse events than the placebo-treated group. According to the Cochrane Database of Systemic Reviews, doses of 16 mg/day were best tolerated when titrated over a 4-week period (54).

Acetylcholinesterase Inhibitors: Additional Considerations

Significant cholinergic side effects occur in up to about 25% of patients receiving higher doses. Often they are related to the initial titration of medication. Patients tend to rapidly become tolerant to the adverse events when they occur. Nausea, diarrhea, vomiting, and weight loss are the most common side effects. An increased but modest incidence of anorexia has been a consistent finding across clinical trials and appears to be dose-related. The absolute reported incidence varies from approximately 8% to 25% at the highest doses compared to 3% to 10% in comparable placebo patients. Similarly, there is an increased rate of significant weight loss with higher doses of ChIs compared to placebo patients. The proportion of patients losing greater than 7% of their baseline weight varies from approximately 10% to 24% in the higher doses and from 2% to 10% of the placebo-treated patients.

Few trials have directly compared the different agents. One comparing donepezil and rivastigmine showed more frequent adverse events associated with rivastigmine during the titration phase but similar frequencies as donepezil in the maintenance phase (56). Two clinical trials testing galantamine in MCI showed an increased mortality rate in the galantamine group (1.5%) compared to placebo (0.4%), leading to an FDA alert (http://www. fda.gov/cder/drug/InfoSheets/HCP/galantamineHCP.htm). However, two clinical trials testing donepezil and one with rivastigmine in MCI did not show an increase in mortality compared to placebo (57–59). A donepezil trial in vascular dementia also showed an increased incidence of deaths in one trial (10 vs. 0) but not in two others (60). Uncommonly, the vagotonic effects of ChIs may cause significant bradycardia, and this can be a particular concern to patients with cardiac conduction impairments or sick sinus syndrome. Because gastric acid secretion may be increased with increased cholinergic tone, there may be an increased risk for developing ulcers or gastrointestinal bleeding. Uncommonly, AChEIs may cause bladder outflow obstruction and seizures, exacerbate asthma or obstructive pulmonary disease, and interfere with succinylcholine-like anesthetics. Because of these actions, AChEIs should be used cautiously in patients with significant asthma, chronic obstructive pulmonary disease, cardiac conduction defects, active peptic ulcers, or clinically significant bradycardia or in patients undergoing anesthesia with the use of succinylcholine-type drugs.

Memantine

The N-methyl-D-aspartate (NMDA) receptor, a glutamate receptor subtype, has important effects in learning and memory. Stimulation by the excitatory amino acid glutamate results in long-term potentiation of neuronal activity basic to memory formation (61). There appears to be a decrease in cerebral cortical and hippocampal NMDA receptors in AD. Glycine, acting at an adjoining glycine-B receptor, modulates the effects of glutamate. Memantine is a noncompetitive NMDA receptor antagonist that binds to the NMDA receptor-operated cation channels. By inhibiting calcium ion influx as a result, it may reduce NMDA-mediated excitotoxicity, although there is currently no clinical evidence that memantine prevents or slows neurodegeneration in patients. Memantine also acts as a noncompetitive antagonist at the 5HT-3 receptor, but the clinical significance of this is unknown (62).

The FDA approved memantine for moderate to severe AD in 2003. Three randomized placebo-controlled trials have shown benefits over placebo in moderate or severe AD on several measures. Two studies, one of which evaluated participants who were being treated with donepezil, showed significant improvements on several clinical outcome measures (63,64), but a 6-month trial in moderate to severe AD did not. The third study, conducted in nursing homes in Latvia, showed a significant advantage of memantine over placebo in daily functioning and global impression of change (65). Another 6-month-long placebo-controlled trial in outpatients with moderate to severe disease did not show advantages for memantine (66). Three trials evaluated memantine in mild to moderate AD. Two of the three failed to show advantages for memantine on cognitive, global, functional, or behavioral outcomes (www.forestclinicaltrials.com, unpublished data 99679, data on file, H. Lundbeck A/S, 2004; 67). According to the Cochrane Database of Systemic Reviews, pooled data on memantine in mild to moderate AD showed a marginal beneficial effect at 6 months that was clinically insignificant, with no effect on behavior or activities of daily living (68). Memantine is not FDA approved for mild AD.

Memantine is available in tablet and oral solution form. Treatment is initiated with 5 mg/daily for 1 week, with the dosage increased by 5 mg/daily in divided doses to a maintenance dose of 10 mg twice a day. Side effects can include dizziness, constipation, headache, and confusion. Generally, memantine is well tolerated and is thought to have low potential for drug interactions.

Returning to our illustrative vignettes, any of the cholinesterase inhibitors would be appropriate as monotherapy for the patient in vignette A, while memantine or donepezil would be appropriate choices for the patient in vignette B.

References

1. McKhann G, Drachman D, Folstein M, et al. Clinical diagnosis of Alzheimer's disease: Report of the NINCDS-ADRDA Work Group under the auspices of Department of Health and Human Services Task Force on Alzheimer's Disease. Neurology 1984;34:939–944.

2. Bowen DM, Smith CB, White P, et al. Neurotransmitter-related enzymes and indices of hypoxia in senile dementia and other abiotrophies. Brain 1976;99:459–496.

3. Davies P, Maloney AJ. Selective loss of central cholinergic neurons in Alzheimer's disease [letter]. Lancet 1976;2:1403.

4. Perry EK, Perry RH, Blessed G, et al. Necropsy evidence of central cholinergic deficits in senile dementia. Lancet 1977;1:189.

5. Arendt T, Bigl V, Arendt A, et al. Loss of neurons in the nucleus basalis of Meynert in Alzheimer's disease, paralysis agitans and Korsakoff's disease. Acta Neuropathol 1983;61:101–108.

6. Whitehouse PJ, Price DL, Struble RG, et al. Alzheimer's disease and senile dementia: Loss of neurons in the basal forebrain. Science 1982;215:1237–1239.

7. Arendt T, Bigl V, Tennstedt A, et al. Neuronal loss in different parts of the nucleus basalis is related to neuritic plaque formation in cortical target areas in Alzheimer's disease. Neuroscience 1985;14:1–14.

8. Etienne P, Robitaille Y, Gauthier S, et al. Nucleus basalis neuronal loss and neuritic plaques in advanced Alzheimer's disease. Can J Physiol Pharmacol 1986;64:318–324.

9. Perry EK, Tomlinson BE, Blessed G, et al. Correlation of cholinergic abnormalities with senile plaques and mental test scores in senile dementia. Br Med J 1978;2:1457–1459.

10. Bondareff W, Mountjoy CQ, Roth M. Loss of neurons of origin of the adrenergic projection to cerebral cortex (nucleus locus coeruleus) in senile dementia. Neurology 1982;32:164–168.

11. Mann DM, Yates PO, Marcyniuk B. A comparison of changes in the nucleus basalis and locus coeruleus in Alzheimer's disease. J Neurol Neurosurg Psychiatry 1984;47:201–203.

12. Zubenko GS, Moossy J. Major depression in primary dementia. Clinical and neuropathologic correlates. Arch Neurol 1988;45:1182–1186.

13. Zweig RM, Ross CA, Hedreen JC, et al. The neuropathology of aminergic nuclei in Alzheimer's disease. Ann Neurol 1988;24:233–242.

14. Zubenko GS, Moossy J, Kopp U. Neurochemical correlates of major depression in primary dementia. Arch Neurol 1990;47:209–214.

15. Lane RM, Potkin SG, Enz A. Targeting acetylcholinesterase and butyrylcholinesterase in dementia. Int J Neuropsychopharmacol 2006;9:101–124.

16. Christie JE, Shering A, Ferguson J, et al. Physostigmine and arecoline: Effects of intravenous infusions in Alzheimer presenile dementia. Br J Psychiatry 1981;138:46–50.

17. Davis KL, Mohs RC. Enhancement of memory processes in Alzheimer's disease with multiple-dose intravenous physostigmine. Am J Psychiatry 1982;139:1421–1424.

18. Mohs RC, Davis BM, Johns CA, et al. Oral physostigmine treatment of patients with Alzheimer's disease. Am J Psychiatry 1985;142:28–33.

19. Stern Y, Sano M, Mayeux R. Effects of oral physostigmine in Alzheimer's disease. Ann Neurol 1987;22:306–310.

20. Jorm AF. Effects of cholinergic enhancement therapies on memory function in Alzheimer's disease: A meta-analysis of the literature. Aust N Z J Psychiatry 1986;20:237–240.

21. Antuono PG. Effectiveness and safety of velnacrine for the treatment of Alzheimer's disease. A double-blind, placebo-controlled study. Mentane Study Group. Arch Intern Med 1995;155:1766–1772.

22. Davis KL, Thal LJ, Gamzu ER, et al. A double-blind, placebo-controlled multicenter study of tacrine for Alzheimer's disease. The Tacrine Collaborative Study Group. N Engl J Med 1992;327:1253–1259.

23. Thal LJ, Schwartz G, Sano M, et al. A multicenter double-blind study of controlled-release physostigmine for the treatment of symptoms secondary to Alzheimer's disease. Physostigmine Study Group. Neurology 1996;47:1389–1395.

24. Geldmacher DS. Treatment guidelines for Alzheimer's disease: redefining perceptions in primary care. Prim Care Companion J Clin Psychiatry 2007;9(2).

25. Enz A, Floersheim P. Cholinesterase inhibitors: An overview of their mechanisms of action. In: Becker R, ed. Alzheimer's Disease: From Molecular Biology to Therapy. Boston: Birkhauser, 1997:211–215.

26. Brufani M. Filocamo L. Rational design of new acetylcholinesterase inhibitors. In: Becker R, ed. Alzheimer's Disease: From Molecular Biology to Therapy. Boston: Birkhauser, 1997:171–177.

27. Atack JR, Perry EK, Bonham JR, et al. Molecular forms of acetylcholinesterase and butyrylcholinesterase in the aged human central nervous system. J Neurochem 1986;47:263–277.

28. Arendt T, Bruckner MK, Lange M, et al. Changes in acetylcholinesterase and butyrylcholinesterase in Alzheimer's disease resemble embryonic development—a study of molecular forms. Neurochem Int 1992;21(3):381–396.

29. Rogers SL, Doody RS, Mohs RC, et al. Donepezil improves cognition and global function in Alzheimer's disease: A 15-week, double-blind, placebo-controlled study. Donepezil Study Group. Arch Intern Med 1998;158:1021–1031.

30. Rogers SL, Farlow MR, Doody RS, et al. A 24-week, double-blind, placebo-controlled trial of donepezil in patients with Alzheimer's disease. Donepezil Study Group. Neurology 1998;50:136–145.

31. Burns A, Rossor M, Hecker J, et al. The effects of donepezil in Alzheimer's disease—results from a multinational trial. Dementia Geriatric Cognitive Disorders 1999;10:237–244.

32. Winblad B, Bonura ML, Rossini BM, et al. Nicergoline in the treatment of mild-to-moderate Alzheimer's disease: A European multicentre trial. Clin Drug Invest 2001;21:621–632.

33. Tariot PN, Cummings JL, Katz IR, et al. A randomized, double-blind, placebo-controlled study of the efficacy and safety of donepezil in patients with Alzheimer's disease in the nursing home setting. J Am Geriatr Soc 2001;49(12):1590–1599.

34. Mohs RC, Doody RS, Morris JC, et al. 1-year, placebo-controlled preservation of function survival study of donepezil in AD patients. Neurology 2001;57:481–488.

35. Feldman H, Gauthier S, Hecker J, et al. A 24-week, randomized, double-blind study of donepezil in moderate to severe Alzheimer's disease. Neurology 2001;57:613–620.

36. Winblad B, Kilander L, Eriksson S, et al. Donepezil in patients with severe Alzheimer's disease: Double-blind, parallel-group, placebo-controlled study. [erratum appears in Lancet. 2006 Jan 17;367(9527):1980]. Lancet 2006;367(9516):1057–1065.

37. Homma A, Takeda M, Imai Y, et al. Clinical efficacy and safety of donepezil on cognitive and global function in patients with Alzheimer's disease. A 24-week, multicenter, double-blind, placebo-controlled study in Japan. E2020 Study Group. Dementia Geriatr Cognitive Disorders 2000;11(6):299–313.

38. Courtney C, Farrell D, Gray R, et al. Long-term donepezil treatment in 565 patients with Alzheimer's disease (AD2000): Randomised double-blind trial. Lancet 2004;363(9427):2105–2115.

39. Hashimoto M, Kazui H, Matsumoto K, et al. Does donepezil treatment slow the progression of hippocampal atrophy in patients with Alzheimer's disease? Am J Psychiatry 2005;162(4):676–682.

40. Jack CR Jr, Petersen RC, Grundman M, et al. Longitudinal MRI findings from the vitamin E and donepezil treatment study for MCI. Neurobiol Aging 2008;29:1285–1295.

41. Corey-Bloom J, Anand R, Veach J, et al. A randomized trial evaluating the efficacy and safety of ENA 713 (rivastigmine tartrate): A new acetylcholinesterase inhibitor, in patients with mild to moderately severe Alzheimer's disease. Int J Geriatr Psychopharmacol 1998;1:55–65.

42. Rosler M, Anand R, Cicin-Sain A, et al. Efficacy and safety of rivastigmine in patients with Alzheimer's disease: International randomised controlled trial. Br Med J 1999;318:633–638.

43. Birks J, Grimley Evans J, Iakovidou V, et al. Rivastigmine for Alzheimer's disease. Cochrane Database of Systematic Reviews 2000;(4): CD001191.

44. Schneider L. Rivastigmine. In Qizilbash N, Schneider L, Chui H, et al, eds. Evidence-Based Dementia Practice. Oxford, UK: Blackwell Science, 2002:499–509.

45. Schneider LS, Anand R, Farlow M. Systematic review of the efficacy of rivastigmine for patients with Alzheimer's disease. Int J Geriatr Psychopharmacol 1998;1:S26–S34.

46. Spencer CM, Noble S. Rivastigmine: A review of its use in Alzheimer's disease. Drugs Aging 1998;13:391–411.

47. Winblad B, Cummings J, Andreasen N, et al. A six-month double-blind, randomized, placebo-controlled study of a transdermal patch in Alzheimer's disease–rivastigmine patch versus capsule. Int J Geriatr Psychiatry 2007;22(5):456–467.

48. Harvey AL. The pharmacology of galantamine and its analogues. Pharmacology Therapeutics 1995;68:113–128.

49. Maelicke A, Samochocki M, Jostock R, et al. Allosteric sensitization of nicotinic receptors by galantamine, a new treatment strategy for Alzheimer's disease. Biol Psychiatry 2001;49:279–288.

50. Raskind M, Peskind ER, Wessel T, et al. Galantamine in Alzheimer's disease: a 6-month, randomized, placebo-controlled trial with a 6-month extension. Neurology 2000;54:2261–2268.

51. Tariot PN, Solomon PR, Morris JC, et al. A 5-month, randomized, placebo-controlled trial of galantamine in AD. The Galantamine USA-10 Study Group. Neurology 2000;54:2269–2276.

52. Wilcock GK, Lilienfeld S, Gaens E. Efficacy and safety of galantamine in patients with mild to moderate Alzheimer's disease: Multicentre randomised controlled trial. Galantamine International-1 Study Group. Br Med J 2000;321:1445–1449.

53. Rockwood K, Mintzer J, Truyen L, et al. Effects of a flexible galantamine dose in Alzheimer's disease: A randomised, controlled trial. J Neurol Neurosurg Psychiatry 2001;71:589–595.

54. Loy C, Schneider L. Galantamine for Alzheimer's disease and mild cognitive impairment. Cochrane Database of Systematic Reviews 2006;(1): CD001747.

55. Brodaty H, Corey-Bloom J, Potocnik FC, et al. Galantamine prolonged-release formulation in the treatment of mild to moderate Alzheimer's disease. Dementia Geriatr Cognitive Disorders 2005;20(2–3):120–132.

56. Bullock R, Touchon J, Bergman H, et al. Rivastigmine and donepezil treatment in moderate to moderately severe Alzheimer's disease over a 2-year period. Curr Med Res Opin 2005;21(8):1317–1327.

57. Salloway S, Ferris S, Kluger A et al. Efficacy of donepezil in mild cognitive impairment: A randomized placebo-controlled trial. Neurology 2004;63:651–657.

58. Petersen RC, Thomas RG, Grundman M et al. Alzheimer's Disease Cooperative Study Group. Vitamin E and donepezil for the treatment of mild cognitive impairment. N Engl J Med 2005;352:2379–2388.

59. Feldman HH, Ferris S, Winblad B, et al. Effect of rivastigmine on delay to diagnosis of Alzheimer's disease from mild cognitive impairment: The InDDEx study. Lancet Neurol 2007;6(6):501–512.

60. Kavirajan H, Schneider LN. Efficacy and adverse effects of cholinesterase inhibitors and memantine in vascular dementia: A meta-analysis of randomized controlled trials. Lancet Neurol 2007;6(9):782–792.

61. Cotman CW, Monaghan DT, Ganong AH. Excitatory amino acid neurotransmission: NMDA receptors and Hebb-type synaptic plasticity. Ann Rev Neurosci 1988;11:61–80.

62. Rammes G, Rupprecht R, Ferrari U, et al. The N-methyl-D-aspartate receptor channel blockers memantine, MRZ 2/579 and other amino-alkylcyclohexanes antagonise 5-HT(3) receptor currents in cultured HEK-293 and N1E-115 cell systems in a non-competitive manner. Neurosci Lett 2001;306(1–2):81–84.

63. Reisberg B, Doody R, Stoffler A, et al. Memantine in moderate-to severe Alzheimer's disease. N Engl J Med 2003;348(14):1333–1341.

64. Tariot PN, Farlow MR, Grossberg GT, et al. Memantine treatment in patients with moderate to severe Alzheimer disease already receiving donepezil: A randomized controlled trial. JAMA 2004;291(3):317–324.

65. Winblad B, Poritis N. Memantine in severe dementia: Results of the 9M-Best Study (Benefit and efficacy in severely demented patients during treatment with memantine). Int J Geriatr Psychiatry 1999;14:135–146.

66. van Dyck CH, Tariot PN, Meyers B, et al. A 24-week randomized, controlled trial of memantine in patients with moderate-to-severe Alzheimer disease. Alzheimer Dis Assoc Disorders 2007;21(2):136–143.

67. Peskind ER, Potkin SG, Pomara N, et al. Memantine treatment in mild to moderate Alzheimer disease: A 24-week randomized, controlled trial. Am J Geriatr Psychiatry 2006;14(8):704–715.

68. McShane R, Areosa Sastre A, Minakaran N. Memantine for dementia. Cochrane Database Systematic Reviews 2006;(2): CD003154.

Chapter 10

Pharmacotherapy: behavioral problems

Pharmacotherapy of behavioral disorders in patients with dementia is limited to off-label therapy. There are no approved agents for the treatment of agitation, for example, in AD patients. Nonpharmacological management will be discussed later, but it is not universally effective. FDA-approved agents have some modest benefits, but often behavioral problems arise in patients already on such therapy, or they are otherwise inadequately controlled by such therapy. The agents that are used have been chosen on the basis of their proven efficacy in other diseases in the hope that they will be similarly effective in patients whose behavioral disorder results from AD.

Literature reviews suggest that up to 90% of patients with dementia will develop significant behavioral problems at some point in the course of illness (1), while population-based studies suggest that the figure is actually closer to 100% (2). The implication is that "behavioral and psychological signs and symptoms of dementia" (3) are major features of dementia and require a thoughtful appreciation of their phenomenology, assessment, and management. The behavioral changes seen in dementia tend to occur in clusters of signs and symptoms that may vary among patients and within patients over time rather than as syndromes that characterize other psychiatric disorders, presumably reflecting the complex interaction between cognitive deficits and environmental variables. Despite efforts to propose syndromal criteria for "psychosis" (4) and "depression" of AD (5), these proposed criteria have not been validated. We therefore adhere to a rather pragmatic approach of describing an individual patient's clusters of signs and symptoms and using them as guideposts in the selection of appropriate therapy.

Cohen-Mansfield and Billig (6) defined agitation as "inappropriate verbal, vocal, or motor activity unexplained by apparent needs or confusion." This straightforward definition emphasizes the clinician's responsibility first to presume that the behaviors have some meaning, even if not immediately perceptible. Shouting or striking out during care should not be dismissed as "agitation" mandating psychotropic therapy when in fact a specific behavioral intervention might be identified. The following four vignettes illustrate common behavioral symptom clusters that we will use to guide treatment recommendations.

Vignette A: Depression

A 64-year-old woman with MCI (amnestic single domain) has withdrawn from her friends and activities, embarrassed and fearful that her memory loss will cause her to forget friends' names and directions to favorite locales and otherwise impair her social skills. Despite all assurances to the contrary, she fears that her friends pity her and prefer to avoid her. Consequently she sits alone at home while her husband is at work and watches some television but dislikes almost all daytime TV programs. She tries to read but complains she cannot remember the plot, and so she has largely abandoned reading as well. Her husband reports she is often tearful at home, expressing the futility of her life. She is taking donepezil 10 mg daily. Her MMSE score is 26/30, and during her examination she appears overtly depressed.

Vignette B: Anxiety

A 72-year-old woman with mild-stage dementia caused by AD is afraid to let her husband out of her sight. When he closes the bathroom door, she knocks on it until he re-emerges. She takes galantamine 16 mg daily. Her MMSE score, with encouragement, is 23/30. However, with nearly every question she first turns to her husband, who is seated in the room with her, and tells him, "I can't do that." But with further prodding, she usually provides the correct answer. Her husband confides he feels he is succumbing to the extreme stress her continuous anxiety places on him.

Vignette C: Agitation and Aggression

An 82-year-old couple comes to see you because of concerns regarding the husband's "memory." He denies quite vigorously that he has any problem whatsoever, and his wife appears fearful of disagreeing. However, a handwritten note provided by their son describes a number of typical instances of memory loss, as well as major changes in personality. He reports that his father has become very irritable and quick to anger and sometimes will strike others or throw something. For example, when he becomes frustrated while unsuccessfully trying to work the television remote control, he pronounces it broken. If anyone tries to show him, or disagree, he yells and throws it on the floor. On one occasion he threatened to hit his wife when she corrected one of his misstatements about where the children were living. On examination, performed with some difficulty due to poor cooperation, his MMSE score is 21/30. Because his level of cooperation is felt to be poor, he is given the rivastigmine patch and seems to tolerate it well, though most of the time he forgets it is on. Several months later, his wife is brought to the hospital with a traumatic intracranial hemorrhage after he hit her on the head with his cane for trying to tell him he should not drive. Unfortunately, due to the severity of her injury, she herself required discharge to a skilled nursing facility and never fully recovered.

Vignette D: Psychosis

A 75-year-old woman is brought in with a slowly progressive dementia. Over the past 6 months she has become increasingly suspicious that others "have it in" for her and are "ganging up" on her, and that family members are using her prescribed medications to poison her. When family tried to reassure her, she became enraged, shouted accusations, and became physically resistive and combative. Eventually, she developed the intermittent belief that some family members were intruders who intended to kill her, as well as the persistent belief that dead family members were alive and that she could see and communicate with them. She sometimes reported seeing animals in the house and reacted with fear or rage at those times.

A Rational Approach to Evaluation

Articulating a logical approach to the evaluation and management of a clinical dilemma is by itself therapeutic, since it offers reassurance to families and caregivers that a confusing situation can be clarified, understood, and helped. The approach proposed here, summarized in Table 10.1, is an elaboration of prior work (7–10).

Nonpharmacological Interventions

Nonpharmacological interventions can include trying to cue or reorient the person in a manner that is not frustrating; ensuring that the environment is comfortable and permits safe physical activity, while providing visual cues; avoiding excessive stress or demands; maintaining a regular schedule of

Table 10.1 Evaluation and Management Schema

1. Define target symptoms in consensual manner with informants.
2. Establish or revisit medical diagnoses.
3. Establish or revisit neuropsychiatric diagnoses.
4. Assess and reverse aggravating factors.
5. Adapt to specific cognitive deficits.
6. Identify relevant psychosocial factors.
7. Educate caregivers.
8. Employ behavior management principles.
9. Use psychotropics for specific psychiatric syndromes.
10. For remaining problems, consider symptomatic pharmacotherapy:
    - Use psychobehavioral metaphor.
    - Use medication class relevant to metaphor and with empirical evidence of efficacy.
    - "Start low, go slow."
    - Avoid toxicity.
    - Use lowest effective dose.
    - Withdraw after appropriate period and observe for relapse.
    - Serial trials are sometimes needed.

Adapted from Rosenquist K, Tariot P, Loy R. Treatments for behavioural and psychological symptoms in AD and other dementias. In O'Brien J, ed. Dementia. London: Edward Arnold, 2000:571–602.

pleasant events; and optimizing interpersonal variables—for example, simplifying language, avoiding negative statements, and avoiding confrontation (11). Cohen-Mansfield (12) offered an overview of approaches, such as music, pet therapy, massage, recordings of familiar people, walking programs, and the like. Most physicians are not comfortable with these approaches, which do require a degree of familiarity and need to be tailored to each situation. It is therefore extremely helpful to partner with other specialists to assist in formulating a care plan, and to learn how to formulate them more independently over time. The choice of specialist may vary depending upon the community and the specific need; the options can include nurse specialists, social workers, selected psychologists or neuropsychologists, occupational therapists, speech therapists, or physical therapists.

Pharmacological Interventions: General Precepts

There are no FDA-approved treatments for relief of psychopathology associated with dementia, so clinicians must rely on trials data, evidence, and experience. For nonurgent problems where nonpharmacological interventions have been exhausted, we advocate an approach that rests on a description of target symptoms that are analogous to a drug-responsive psychiatric syndrome, termed the "psychobehavioral metaphor" (13). We match dominant target symptoms (i.e., the "metaphor") to the most relevant drug class. While this face-valid approach is reflected in most consensus guidelines (14–17), it has not been established empirically.

In selecting a medication, we prefer those with at least some empirical evidence of efficacy and with the highest likelihood of tolerability and safety. We start with low doses and escalate slowly, assessing target symptoms as well as toxicity. We discontinue the medication if it is harmful or ineffective. If a psychotropic is helpful at subtoxic doses, an empirical trial is often performed in reverse after a period of stability, monitoring the patient closely for re-emergence of the problem. This very approach is mandated in the nursing home setting by federal regulations created in 1987. Occasionally we try several different medications before a useful one is identified; sometimes combinations are considered, despite the complete absence of prospective clinical trials data to guide this approach. However, sometimes no medication is found that is helpful. This sobering reality underscores the importance of deploying non-medication approaches first and foremost.

Depression

Depressive features in AD patients not only add to caregiver concern but also materially reduce the functionality and quality of life of the patient. Effective treatment of depression in a patient with dementia can have a greater impact on cognitive and functional abilities than cholinesterase inhibitors and memantine.

The anticholinergic side effects of older agents, particularly the tricyclic antidepressants, risk exacerbating confusion and are often intolerable; this makes them a poor choice for depression management in AD patients who have reduced cerebral acetylcholine and are often receiving cholinesterase inhibitor therapy. Tricyclics are often prescribed for other purposes, such as sleep and pain control, and should be avoided in all of these contexts in AD patients unless there is a compelling reason to maintain them.

As a drug class, the selective serotonin reuptake inhibitors (SSRIs) have a generally more favorable side effect profile. Evidence for antidepressant efficacy in patients with dementia is weak, but this class is nonetheless preferred (18–20). In some cases, they may also ease agitation, but they are not sufficiently effective for acute intervention for severe agitation. SSRIs occasionally precipitate REM sleep behavior disorder, and this may in turn suggest an underlying synucleinopathy such as dementia with Lewy bodies. If this becomes problematic, discontinuing or changing the SSRI should be considered (21).

In patients with depressive features who are also having trouble sleeping, the use of a sedating antidepressant, such as trazodone or mirtazapine, at bedtime could be considered, though randomized controlled trials are lacking (22,23).

Anxiety

Anxious features are common among patients with dementia and as illustrated in vignette B can manifest with excessive dependency on the caregiver, even to the point of not letting him or her out of sight. This is uncomfortable for the patient and can quickly wear down the caregiver. SSRIs are usually selected first; if ineffective, short-acting benzodiazepines such as lorazepam can be considered. There is no evidence supporting the use of buspirone in dementia, but it is sometimes considered.

Agitation, Aggression, and Psychosis

Psychosis with or without agitation and aggression can be an urgent and dangerous problem, as illustrated in vignettes C and D. If an emergency arises in which there is a real consideration of physical harm, hospitalization and/or antipsychotic administration should be the first-line options considered (Fig. 10.1). Psychotic features include hallucinations (typically but not exclusively visual, especially in patients with dementia with Lewy bodies) and delusions, often paranoid in nature, and can be associated with agitation that in turn can lead to violence. Psychosis with agitation and agitation that jeopardizes the well-being of the patient or caregiver therefore require timely and effective treatment.

Given the state of the literature, the clinician confronted by a psychotic demented patient is asked to steer a difficult course between the real risk of harm in the absence of definitely effective therapy and the admonitions regarding off-label use, treatment-related adverse effects, and potential inefficacy from the medical literature. Any advice in this setting is susceptible to valid criticism. With these strong caveats in mind, here is ours.

Sink et al (20) reviewed controlled trials or meta-analyses of medications used to treat varying types of psychopathology, including agitation and psychosis. They, and others, concluded that the most consistent evidence for efficacy has been found with antipsychotics. Within the context of the "metaphor"

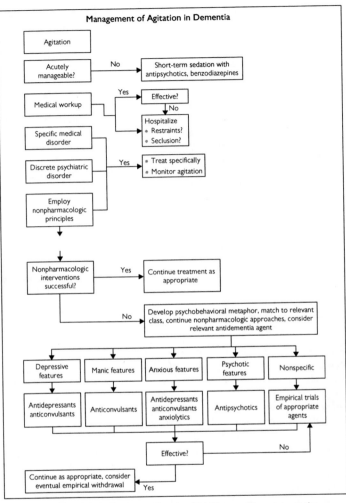

Management of Agitation in Dementia

Figure 10.1 Dementia and Violence: Caregiver Risk 82 year old woman was the caregiver of her demented husband until he hit her on the head with a metal cane. She was discharged to a nursing home with severe post-traumatic cognitive impairment. Adapted from Tariot. J Clin Pssychiatry. 1999;60(suppl 8):11–20 ©.

approach, antipsychotics would be used first for treatment of agitation with psychotic features, but in fact antipsychotics are prescribed and have been studied in a wide array of forms of psychopathology.

There are two main classes of antipsychotics: so-called conventional antipsychotics and the newer atypical agents. Lanctot et al (24) performed a meta-analysis of studies of conventional agents and reported an average therapeutic effect (antipsychotic vs. placebo) of 26%, with placebo response rates ranging from 19% to 50%. Side effects were reported to occur more often on drug than placebo (mean difference 25%). Side effects are common, including akathisia, parkinsonism, tardive dyskinesia, sedation, peripheral and central anticholinergic effects, postural hypotension, cardiac conduction defects, and falls (23). For these reasons, there was great hope that atypical antipsychotics would have special utility in patients with dementia (15,17).

Regarding atypicals, the meta-analysis of Schneider et al (25) is most helpful, partly because it included results from 15 published as well as publicly presented but not published placebo-controlled studies of atypical antipsychotics, the latter including trials that had been completed years ago. The trials generally lasted a few weeks and included participants with dementia of varying types complicated by agitation and/or aggression and/or psychosis. Altogether, 3,353 patients received medication and 1,757 received placebo. The results showed an incremental treatment benefit of about 18% for active drug over placebo—that is, about 1 in 5 patients in these trials experienced significant improvement in symptoms. Atypical antipsychotics were about three times as likely as placebo to cause adverse events, the most common being somnolence, falls with and without injury, syncope, parkinsonism, bruising, peripheral edema, and infections.

Cerebrovascular adverse events have been seen in about 1.9% of those receiving atypical antipsychotics versus 0.9% of those receiving placebo, resulting in an FDA safety warning for the use of aripiprazole, risperidone, and olanzapine in this population. Subsequent studies have found no increased risk of stroke between atypical and typical antipsychotics, meaning that merely switching classes is not likely to confer benefit in this respect. Further, the death rate in clinical trials was 3.5% with atypicals versus 2.3% with placebo, leading the FDA to impose a "black-box" warning at first for all atypicals, and then later for all antipsychotics as a class based on subsequent studies involving large public databases that found a similar rate of deaths among elderly people receiving typical antipsychotics.

The Clinical Antipsychotic Trials of Intervention Effectiveness—Alzheimer's Disease (CATIE-AD) effectiveness trial attempted to address an issue not previously investigated: the comparative utility of commonly used atypicals (26). Patients with AD and psychosis, aggression, or agitation were randomly assigned to treatment with olanzapine, quetiapine, risperidone, or placebo. The primary measure of effectiveness was time to all-cause discontinuation; however, there was no significant difference among the treatment conditions (Table 10.2). The basic conclusion of the study was that a limited number of patients receive benefit without being harmed: these are the patients for whom continued therapy is rational.

The literature and our own clinical experience suggest that atypical antipsychotic agents are the preferred agents (especially in patients with parkinsonism) because they can be effective and are less likely to cause or exacerbate extrapyramidal syndromes in comparison to the typical agents. Quetiapine in

Table 10.2 CATIE-AD Trial Key Findings

Discontinuation Reason	Olanzepine (n = 99)	Quetiapine (n = 94)	Risperidone (n = 84)	Placebo (n = 139)	P*
Any cause, median, wk	8.1	5.3	7.4	8.0	0.52
Lack of efficacy, median, wk	22.1	9.1	26.7	9.0	0.002
Intolerability, adverse events, or death, % pts	24%	16%	18%	5%	0.009
Improvement on CGIC scale, % pts	32%	26%	29%	21%	0.22

*For time to discontinuation of overall treatment group vs. placebo.

Based on Schneider LS, Tariot PN, Dagerman KS, et al. effectiveness of atypical antipsychotic drugs in patients with Alzheimer's disease. N Engl J Med 2006;355:1525–1538.

particular has minimal to no extrapyramidal effects. Older agents (the "typical" antipsychotic drugs such as haloperidol) are effective but have a high likelihood of causing or exacerbating parkinsonism and a much higher risk of tardive dyskinesia if used chronically. All antipsychotics carry a significant risk of sedation. Mortality associated with neuroleptic use in the older dementia population is higher in those treated with conventional neuroleptics compared to the newer atypical neuroleptics (27). Therefore, the use of atypical neuroleptics requires that the patient's family and other physicians involved in a patient's care feel that the benefits outweigh the risks. As with all psychoactive medications, care must be used and the dose and duration of use minimized.

Figure 10.1 summarizes our approach to the management of patients with agitation.

Other Psychotropics

Other options that are sometimes used include valproic acid, trazodone, and SSRIs. These can show efficacy in individual patients, despite the discouraging trials data; however, the apparently lesser concern about safety by virtue of lack of analogous black box warnings is misleading, since there have not been sufficiently large trials to establish whether there is in fact less risk in using these agents.

The study by Sink et al (20) found little evidence of efficacy of antidepressants for treating neuropsychiatric symptoms other than depression. Since depressive features are common in patients with dementia and frequently include irritability, serotonergic antidepressants are used commonly in practice. Sink et al (20) also found lack of support for the use of divalproex and mixed results regarding the efficacy of carbamazepine in patients with dementia. In practice, these are sometimes used when more conventional approaches fail. Practice guidelines have endorsed these approaches, even in the absence of convincing evidence (17).

Acetylcholinesterase inhibitors (28) and memantine (29) may also have behavior-modifying effects, and for the occasional patient not yet receiving these agents, their use should be considered for nonemergent behavioral problems. Many patients with dementia, however, who develop behavioral problems are already on these medications.

Sink et al (20) reported that cholinesterase inhibitors had a small but statistically significant benefit for behavioral symptoms, but memantine had no significant benefit. A meta-analysis by Trinh et al (30) also reported a slight overall benefit of cholinesterase inhibitors in patients with mild to moderate AD. More recently, Doody et al (31) reported a meta-analysis of the behavioral effects of memantine, suggesting an overall modest benefit. Our view is that best practice includes routine use of antidementia therapies in most patients with AD as well as certain other dementias, so that psychotropic use usually occurs against this backdrop.

Since clinical trials of all of these agents were aimed toward obtaining regulatory approval and not informing clinical practice, evidence is not available guiding best practice for issues such as the choice of one agent versus the other for relief of behavioral symptoms, or of using psychotropics in combination with these agents. As is often the case, practice will outstrip evidence for the foreseeable future. In the field, (1) inaction is not an option, (2) anecdotal experiences contradict published research, and (3) efficacy has been demonstrated in nondemented patient cohorts.

Other Behavioral Issues

Among patients with executive or behavioral variant AD, other behavioral symptoms that may be more characteristic of frontotemporal dementia also occur. Apathy may be the single most common behavioral disorder affecting these patients. It may be more distressing to caregivers than to patients and is rarely a cause for behavioral intervention. Although perceived as behavioral, one could argue it is as much intellectual, representing a paucity of spontaneous ideation and motivation, cognitively oriented functions generally attributed to frontal networks. Cholinesterase inhibitors may modestly ameliorate apathy as measured by behavioral inventories such as the Neuropsychiatric Inventory (31,32). Perseveration, another manifestation of frontal lobe dysfunction, can be regarded as either a behavioral problem or a manifestation of intellectual impairment (getting "stuck in set"). Either way, this can lead to distressing outcomes, such as the repetitive purchase, collection, and hoarding of magazines or other objects; repetitive gestures or activities or requests; and persistent attempts at some undesired behavior (taking out the trash when there is none to take out, for example). There is no highly effective pharmacotherapeutic intervention, and in extreme cases it may be treated with neuroleptics, although there is no specific "anti-perseveration" effect, but rather a general reduction in spontaneity, thereby exacerbating apathy and inertia.

Returning to our vignettes, initial treatment options for the depressed patient in vignette A include any of the SSRIs. Concomitant use of an acetylcholinesterase inhibitor or memantine is not usually a problem. Similarly, the anxious patient in vignette B would most likely be given an SSRI. A benzodiazepine or buspirone would be a distant second choice. If they prove to be ineffective, consideration could be given to an atypical antipsychotic such as quetiapine, but bearing in mind the risk associated with this choice. The patients in vignettes C and D require something considerably more effective than an acetylcholinesterase inhibitor. While some might advocate the addition of memantine, the outcome of his unfortunate wife illustrates all too clearly how serious such behavior can become, and consideration of an agent with proven efficacy for agitation and psychosis is warranted. While some studies have raised doubts as to their efficacy in the setting of dementia, there is no doubt in the setting of primary psychotic disorders, and many behavioral neurologists and geropsychiatrists use these agents in dementia patients as well. Quetiapine tends to be the best tolerated (little to no extrapyramidal effect) but is not always effective. Risperidone (and haloperidol) is also sometimes efficacious but more likely to have extrapyramidal effects.

References

1. Tariot PN, Blazina L. The psychopathology of dementia. In Morris J, ed. Handbook of Dementing Illnesses. New York: Marcel Dekker Inc., 1993:461–475.

2. Lyketsos CG, Sheppard JM, Steele CD, et al. Randomized, placebo-controlled, double-blind clinical trial of sertraline in the treatment of depression complicating Alzheimer's disease: initial results from the Depression in Alzheimer's Disease study. Am J Psychiatry 2000;157:1686–1689.

3. Finkel SI, Costa e Silva J, Cohen G, et al. Behavioral and psychological signs and symptoms of dementia: a consensus statement on current knowledge and implications for research and treatment. Int Psychogeriatrics 1996;8(suppl 3):497–500.

4. Jeste DV, Finkel SI. Psychosis of Alzheimer's disease and related dementias. Diagnostic criteria for a distinct syndrome. Am J Geriatr Psychiatry 2000;8:29–34.

5. Olin JT, Fox LS, Pawluczyk S, et al. A pilot randomized trial of carbamazepine for behavioral symptoms in treatment-resistant outpatients with Alzheimer's disease Am J Geriatr Psychiatry 2001;9:400–405.

6. Cohen-Mansfield J, Billig N. Agitated behaviors in the elderly. I. A conceptual review. J Am Geriatr Soc 1986;34:711–721.

7. Tariot PN. Treatment strategies for agitation and psychosis in dementia. J Clin Psychiatry 1996;57(suppl 14):21–29.

8. Tariot PN. Treatment of agitation in dementia. J Clin Psychiatry 1999;60(suppl 8): 11–20.

9. Rosenquist K, Tariot P, Loy R. Treatments for behavioural and psychological symptoms in AD and other dementias. In O'Brien J, ed. Dementia. London: Edward Arnold, 2000:571–602.

10. Profenno LA, Tariot PN. Pharmacologic management of agitation in Alzheimer's disease. Dement Geriatr Cogn Disord 2000;17:65–77.

11. Lyketsos CG, Colenda CC, Beck C, et al. Position statement of the American Association for Geriatric Psychiatry regarding principles of care for patients with dementia resulting from Alzheimer disease. Am J Geriatr Psychiatry 2006;14:561–572.

12. Cohen-Mansfield J. Nonpharmacologic interventions for inappropriate behaviors in dementia: A review and critique. Am J Geriatr Psychiatry 2001;9:361–381.

13. Leibovici A, Tariot PN. Agitation associated with dementia: a systematic approach to treatment. Psychopharmacol Bull 1988;24:49–53.

14. Rabins P, Blacker D, Bland W, et al, American Psychiatric Association Work Group on Alzheimer's Disease and Related Dementias. Practice guideline for the treatment of patients with Alzheimer's disease and other dementias of late life. Am J Psychiatry 1997;154:1–39.

15. Alexopoulos GS, Silver JM, Kahn DA, et al. Treatment of agitation in older persons with dementia. Postgrad Med 1998;April:1–88.

16. Doody RS, Stevens JC, Beck C, et al. Practice parameter: Management of dementia (an evidence-based review). Report of the Quality Standards Subcommittee of the American Academy of Neurology. Neurology 2001;56:1154–1166.

17. Alexopoulos GS, Jeste DV, Chung H, et al. The expert consensus guideline series: treatment of dementia and its behavioral disturbances. Postgrad Med 2005;Spec No:6–22.

18. Tune LE. Depression and Alzheimer's disease. Depress Anxiety 1998;8(suppl 1): 91–95.

19. Lyketsos CG, DelCampo L, Sternberg M, et al. Treating depression in Alzheimer disease: efficacy and safety of sertraline therapy, and the benefits of depression reduction: the DIADS. Arch Gen Psychiatry 2003;60:737–746.

20. Sink KM, Holden KF, Yaffe K. Pharmacological treatment of neuropsychiatric symptoms of dementia. JAMA 2005;293:596–608.

21. Schenck CH, Mahowald MW, Kim SW, et al. Prominent eye movements during NREM sleep and REM sleep behavior disorder associated with fluoxetine treatment of depression and obsessive-compulsive disorder. Sleep 1992;15:226–235.

22. Wiegand MH. Antidepressants for the treatment of insomnia: a suitable approach? Drugs 2008;68:2411–2417.

23. Devanand DP. Behavioral complications and their treatment in Alzheimer's disease. Geriatrics 1997;52(suppl 2):S37–39.

24. Lanctot KL, Best TS, Mittmann N, et al. Efficacy and safety of neuroleptics in behavioral disorders associated with dementia. J Clin Psychiatry 1998;59:550–561.

25. Schneider LS, Dagerman K, Insel PS. Efficacy and adverse effects of atypical antipsychotics for dementia: meta-analysis of randomized, placebo-controlled trials. Am J Geriatr Psychiatry 2006;14:191–210.

26. Schneider LS, Tariot PN, Dagerman KS, et al. effectiveness of atypical antipsychotic drugs in patients with Alzheimer's disease. N Engl J Med 2006;355:1525–1538.

27. Wang PS, Schneeweiss S, Avorn J, et al. Risk of death in elderly users of conventional vs. atypical antipsychotic medications. N Engl J Med 2005;353:2335–2341.

28. Cummings JL, McRae T, Zhang R, et al. Effects of donepezil on neuropsychiatric symptoms in patients with dementia and severe behavioral disorders. Am J Geriatr Psychiatry 2006;14:605–612.

29. Cummings JL, Schneider E, Tariot PN, et al. Behavioral effects of memantine in Alzheimer disease patients receiving donepezil treatment. Neurology 2006; 67:57–63.

30. Trinh NH, Hoblyn J, Mohanty S, Yaffe K. Efficacy of cholinesterase inhibitors in the treatment of neuropsychiatric symptoms and functional impairment in Alzheimer disease: a meta-analysis. JAMA 2003;289:210–216.

31. Doody RS, Tariot PN, Pfeiffer E, et al. Meta-analysis of six-month trials in Alzheimer's disease. Alzheimers Dement 2007;3:7–17.

32. Cummings JL, Mackell J, Kaufer D. Behavioral effects of current Alzheimer's disease treatments: a descriptive review. Alzheimers Dement 2008;4:49–60.

Chapter 11

Pharmacotherapy: other issues

The goal of therapy in patients with AD and any form of dementia is to maximize their quality of life and minimize caregiver burden. In addition to the cognitive and behavioral strategies discussed, other issues may arise in patients that also represent treatment challenges and opportunities. Three categories of such issues are sleep disturbances, comorbid symptoms, and abrupt decline.

Sleep Disturbances

Of the many possible sleep disorders that can affect patients with dementia, the following four are perhaps the most frequently troublesome.

Vignette A: Insomnia

A 79-year-old woman with moderate-stage dementia goes to bed at 9 p.m. and falls asleep readily but wakens initially at midnight to go the bathroom. She may then dress for the day and wake her husband to ask about their plans. On occasion, she has gone out of the house, and once became lost and was brought home by the police. Her husband now gets up every few hours to check on her and has discovered that even after returning to bed, she arises four times a night to go to the bathroom. During the day, she naps while he shops, cleans, pays bills, and cooks. He is becoming exhausted from lack of sleep, and his daughter expresses concern about his health.

Sleep disturbances are common in AD patients, affecting over 40% of patients (1). They are a major stress for caregivers (2) and a frequent reason for institutionalization (3). Patients who either have trouble falling asleep or else wake up very early and will not go back to sleep sometimes can be helped with nonpharmacological interventions. Daytime napping of no more than 30 minutes and not later than 1 p.m., daily exercise with greater light exposure (walking outside) for up to 30 minutes, and lightbox exposure for up to an hour daily while indoors can improve nighttime sleep patterns (4). When this fails, a short-acting sedative-hypnotic such as zolpidem or zaleplon can be effective; it can be given either at bedtime or when the patient wakens in the night (5). Antihistamines are not generally recommended because of their lack of established efficacy and their side effect profile (6,7).

Vignette B: REM Sleep Behavior Disorder (RBD)

A 76-year-old man is brought for an evaluation by his wife because of impaired memory and a slowed, shuffling gait that gradually developed over the past 2 years. You notice a bruise on his head and learn that sometimes he acts quite violently in his sleep; he recently fell out of bed. He also carries on conversations in his sleep that are quite clearly articulated, making his wife wonder whether he is really asleep (but he is).

Patients with RBD have dream enactment behavior associated with a loss of muscle atonia on polysomnographic electromyographic recordings due to involvement of cholinergic brain stem nuclei within the context of a synucleinopathy, particularly dementia with Lewy bodies (8). This can be difficult to treat, but some clinicians have advocated the use of low-dose clonazepam (9), while monitoring patients carefully for any benzodiazepine-related exacerbation in cognitive impairment or ataxia. There are anecdotal reports of occasional efficacy with melatonin, an inexpensive and generally well-tolerated over-the-counter agent.

Vignette C: Obstructive Sleep Apnea (OSA)

An obese 64-year-old businessman with a family history of dementia reports he is having trouble with his memory. He feels less attentive and is tired all the time and unable to concentrate. His wife reports that he snores a great deal, and within the past year he once fell asleep briefly while driving. He scores 29/30 on the MMSE.

OSA should be suspected in any overweight patient complaining of daytime somnolence. In patients with OSA and mild cognitive difficulties, treating underlying OSA can sometimes improve the cognitive syndrome. OSA is not a cause of dementia but can be a cause of mild cognitive complaints that may be mistaken for early-stage AD (10). It is also found more commonly in persons with APOE e4 (11,12), which is in turn a risk factor for AD and is commonly found in AD patients. Overnight oximetry is a simple screening test showing a sawtooth pattern of oxygen desaturation during sleep, but if OSA is truly suspected, a formal sleep study should be performed. If confirmed, treatment with continuous positive airway pressure (CPAP) may relieve the daytime somnolence and improve (or at least stabilize) the mild cognitive symptoms.

Nocturia

Though not a primary sleep disorder, this is a common reason some patients with dementia are up at night and tired during the day. Treatment options are similar to those for incontinence, as described below. The first step is to determine whether the cause is a spastic or flaccid bladder. For the former, careful use of a peripherally acting anticholinergic agent such as oxybutynin or tolterodine may be helpful. If the latter, a consultation with a urologist should be arranged, and depending on the cause and severity, intermittent catheterization may be needed.

Comorbid Symptoms

While almost any medical illness can complicate the course of a patient with dementia, there are a few common comorbidities that eventually complicate the course of many or even most patients.

Vignette D: Parkinsonism

An 88-year-old man has severe dementia caused by AD but sleeps well and has no behavioral problems. He has developed a mildly stooped posture and a mildly shuffling gait over the past year. On examination, he scores 0/30 on the MMSE and has a mild rest tremor affecting the right thumb. He can arise from a seated position without assistance and seems steady when he walks despite a mildly stooped posture and slight festination when he starts to walk. His son asks whether his father should take any medication for this apparent parkinsonism.

Mild parkinsonism can be an important diagnostic sign of dementia with Lewy bodies and related disorders, especially when it occurs early in the course of dementia. However, in late-stage dementia, parkinsonian signs are common. In fact, the three most prevalent neuropathological comorbidities in very aged brains are Alzheimer's, Parkinson's, and vascular pathologies, so it is not surprising that parkinsonism may emerge in the setting of advanced neurodegenerative dementia in patients who are typically quite elderly.

Intervention with dopaminergic medications can create or worsen psychotic symptoms, particularly visual hallucinations in vulnerable patients. Treatment should therefore be reserved for those with clinically significant parkinsonism, especially if balance becomes impaired so that falls become a threat. The patient in vignette D has advanced dementia but otherwise seems to be doing about as well as one might hope under the care of his son. He sleeps well and has no behavioral problems. Now he is manifesting parkinsonism but does not seem to be at any imminent risk because his symptoms are mild. Nontreatment in this setting seems most appropriate.

An arguably related condition, normal-pressure hydrocephalus (NPH), has gained recognition by the clinical triad of dementia, gait apraxia, and incontinence. This triad is not unique to NPH and occurs eventually in many patients with dementia. NPH is an important diagnostic consideration since it can sometimes be reversed; it should not be confused with an "end-stage brain" manifesting the same triad for very different reasons.

Urinary Incontinence

In the absence of an obvious cause such as a urinary tract infection (see abrupt decline section), two of the more common causes of urinary frequency and incontinence in patients with dementia are flaccid distended bladders that cause overflow incontinence, and spastic bladders. They can be distinguished by checking a urinary postvoid residual. The former is treated with intermittent catheterization. The latter can usually be managed with peripherally acting anticholinergic agents such as oxybutynin and tolterodine. These risk exacerbating confusion, so care must be taken; however, if started at low doses and titrated gradually, they can often be used safely and effectively. Because of other common illnesses, such as prostate cancer, urological consultation should be considered if there is any question about the etiology of incontinence.

Dysphagia

One of the ways patients with dementia can die is through the eventual failure of swallowing, with resultant aspiration or starvation. Dysphagia arises late in the course of AD, heralding what could be considered its "terminal stage." At this point patients are usually unaware of their surroundings, are uncommunicative, and have long since become wholly dependent on others for all their activities of daily living. At this stage, a decision must be made in which family members must choose between comfort care (withholding oral nutrition, usually in the context of hospice care, with comfort provided until death ensues as an expected outcome) or some form of definitive intervention, typically a percutaneous gastrostomy. In our experience, the overwhelming majority of families opt for the former course, but not without exception. The decision is ultimately a personal one. The clinician's role, at a minimum, is to inform the family of this issue before it results in an unexpected and unwanted emergency room visit following an aspiration event so that a definitive plan may be made in the patient's best interests.

Other Physical Symptoms

The syndromes of AD include MCI, Alzheimer's dementia, and the variant syndromes of visual variant (or posterior cortical atrophy), aphasia, apraxia, and executive dysfunction. The somatic manifestations of the variant syndromes are not generally responsive to medications, but appropriate physical/occupational therapy and safety interventions should be addressed.

Abrupt Decline

Vignette E: Urosepsis

You last saw this 84-year-old woman with mild dementia 2 weeks ago, at which time she had no behavioral or sleeping difficulties, was taking donepezil in addition to her blood pressure medication under her husband's supervision, and was quite upbeat. She scored 22/30 on the MMSE and seemed fine until last night, when her husband reports she was incontinent of urine in bed. This morning he had trouble waking her, and when he did, she was very confused and her speech was garbled and nonsensical. She was unsteady and almost fell several times, so he drove her to the emergency room. She was found to be mildly febrile, with an elevated white blood cell count and a urinary tract infection. In addition to the above features, on examination she now scores 11/30 on the MMSE. Her husband is wondering why her dementia is so much worse today.

Over the protracted course of AD, many patients have times when their dementia seems to be suddenly exacerbated, with greatly increased confusion, slurred speech, somnolence, agitation, tremulousness, unsteadiness, falls, and worsened incontinence. Often this is due to a superimposed illness, typically an infection (urinary tract and pneumonia most commonly), a medication error, an injury of some type, or some other cause that must be sought with a thorough evaluation (Fig. 11.1).

Environmental factors, such as an unusually crowded and chaotic family gathering, as often happens during holidays, can also precipitate or aggravate preexisting behavioral difficulties.

A special category of abrupt decline is delirium that occurs within the context of hospitalization, including postoperative delirium. Among elderly patients, pre-existing dementia increases the risk for delirium in this setting by five- to nine-fold (13–15), and a rough approximation (further influenced by other comorbid conditions) is that an elderly patient with dementia entering the hospital has about a 50% chance of developing postoperative delirium (16). In a study that compared 50 patients with incident delirium to 179 without, delirium increased length of stay (12.1 vs. 7.2 days), hospital mortality (8% vs. 1%), and the rate of posthospital institutionalization (16% vs. 3%) (17). Delirium does not always resolve upon hospital discharge. Among patients who develop delirium during their hospitalization, it will remain in one third at 3 months (18). Over a year of follow-up, 83% of patients discharged with delirium are admitted to a nursing home or die (19), and the cumulative 1-year mortality is 39% (18).

Over the course of a year, the average cost of care for a patient who developed delirium during a hospitalization was 2.5 times higher than an age-matched control. Translating this to real dollars, the total cost estimates attributable to delirium are between $16,303 and $64,421 per patient. As a country, this adds between $38 billion and $152 billion to our national health care bill (20). If these

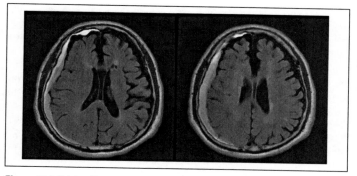

Figure 11.1 Subdural hematoma in an 83 year old man with executive variant Alzheimer's disease (note bifrontal atrophy) causing subacute decline in gait and cognition.

numbers are not sufficiently compelling, consider that as baby boomers enter their retirement years, these numbers can be expected to triple by 2050.

Preventing delirium is the ideal (21). Daily monitoring of cognitive status is the first step so as to know whether a patient is deteriorating or improving. A fast assessment tool is the Benton Orientation Questionnaire (22), which is simply quantification of date and time responses. Patients lose 10 points for each year they are off, 5 points for each month, 1 point for each day of the month, 1 point for each day of the week, and 1 point for each half hour of the time. Anything more than 3 points off is considered abnormal, although in a hospital setting, it is even more important to note the daily trend. To state the obvious, a patient who seems normal but has worsening scores should be viewed as someone with impending delirium, while improving scores in a patient who has been delirious may indicate that he or she is getting better (usually due to treatment he or she is receiving).

For diagnosing delirium, the Confusional Assessment Method (CAM) criteria provide a standardized rating that has been validated with a sensitivity of 94% to 100%, a specificity of 90% to 95%, and high interobserver reliability when conducted by trained research interviewers (23). Diagnosis of delirium requires an acute onset and fluctuating course, inattention (or easy distractibility), and either disorganized thought (manifested by incoherent speech, for example) or an altered level of consciousness (or both).

Nonpharmacological steps that target risk factors can reduce the incidence of postoperative delirium compared with usual care (32% vs. 50%) (24). Such measures include therapeutic activities to address cognitive impairment, physical activity to prevent immobilization, prevention of sleep deprivation, prevention of sensory deprivation by restoring adaptive devices such as eyeglasses and hearing aids, preventing dehydration, and other measures to avoid the addition of psychoactive medications. There is no currently accepted pharmacotherapeutic method for prevention, but in a study of elderly patients presenting with hip fracture, preoperative treatment with low-dose haloperidol reduced the duration and severity of postoperative delirium (25). The absolute incidence was also lower, but the difference did not reach statistical significance. Another study found that a single 1-mg sublingual dose of risperidone immediately following cardiac surgery resulted in a reduced incidence of postoperative delirium (11.1% vs. 31.7%) (26).

If preventive measures fail, the first step is an aggressive search for a reversible cause such as an infection, medication, or electrolyte disturbance, followed by targeted intervention to address the identified cause. However, in many patients no answer is immediately forthcoming, and many require behavioral management for safety reasons regardless of etiology. Pharmacotherapeutic interventions generally rely upon neuroleptic administration, including haloperidol and atypical antipsychotic agents; the lowest effective dose possible should be used (21).

The patient in vignette E has a urinary tract infection and based on her fever, elevated white blood cell count, and delirium may be septic. This is not an exacerbation of AD but a superimposed process, and her husband should be reassured that appropriate antibiotic treatment will result in resolution of the infection and restoration of her pre-infection baseline. The rate of cognitive restoration varies, and while some improvement should occur within days, complete (or nearly complete) recovery can take weeks in some patients.

Prevention

While still not within the current purview of evidence-based clinical practice, the question of prevention frequently arises.

Vignette F: Primary Prevention

A 46-year-old engineer is currently asymptomatic but expresses concern because he has a family history of AD in his mother and maternal grandfather, both of who were diagnosed around age 75 years. He wants to know what he can do to reduce his own risk of developing it. Preventing the onset of the disease is "primary prevention."

Vignette G: Secondary Prevention

Our 46-year-old engineer's mother was diagnosed with AD at age 75 years, and she is now 76 years old. In addition, she has hypothyroidism and diabetes mellitus type 2, both of which require medication. She also had breast cancer 4 years earlier that was locally invasive; she was treated with lumpectomy, local radiation, and raloxifene. Her MMSE score has declined over the preceding 12 months from 23/30 to 12/30, and her son is asking if there is anything that can be done to slow the rate of deterioration. Reducing the rate of disease progression is "secondary prevention."

Primary and secondary prevention are not the same thing, but the two are often confused by patients and their families, as well as the lay media. Primary prevention involves the identification of factors that prevent or slow the onset of disease, while secondary prevention means the slowing of progression of established disease. Either could theoretically involve reducing the rate of neurobiological progression, but to date no such intervention has been found that modifies AD onset or progression. (Secondary prevention, at least as regards symptomatic deterioration, however, can be effected through the management of comorbidities.)

Even if a primary prevention therapy proved to be only partially effective, it could have an enormous impact on our public health system. For example, assuming no change in current longevity, a 5-year delay in symptomatic onset could reduce the number of patients in the United States by half. Unfortunately, there are no established primary prevention therapies for the treatment of AD. Several putative agents have undergone randomized clinical trials and failed, including vitamin E (27), B vitamins (folic acid, vitamin B6, and vitamin B12) (28), nonsteroidal anti-inflammatory drugs (29), estrogen replacement therapy (30), and gingko biloba (31).

Epidemiological and other studies have suggested a reduced incidence of dementia related to healthy lifestyle changes, dietary supplements, and medications; these may therefore merit further investigation. Several primary prevention strategies that also may merit further investigation include aerobic exercise (32–37), mental exercise (38–40), the Mediterranean diet (41,42) (with high intake of vegetables, legumes, fruits, cereals, unsaturated fatty acids primarily from olive oil, a moderately high intake of fish, regular but moderate intake of ethanol primarily from wine, and a low intake of meat, poultry, and dairy products), moderate amounts of ethanol or red wine (43) (which have led some to investigate the amyloid-modifying effects of resveratrol in grapes), foods or dietary supplements containing curcumin (44), vitamin C (45), flavonoids (46,47), and omega-3 fatty acids (48). Lower caloric intake (with reduction in body mass index) has been associated with greater longevity generally, and in APOE e4 carriers (but not noncarriers) a reduced risk of AD (49). The influence of statins and possibly other lipid-lowering agents on AD risk and progression remains controversial, with conflicting conclusions from both epidemiological (50,51) and clinical (52,53) studies. Evidence that rosiglitazone, an insulin-sensitizing agent, may slow AD progression comes from in vitro studies (54,55), animal models (56), and epidemiological (57,58) and clinical studies (59,60) that await further clinical confirmation.

Secondary prevention, as defined by mitigating symptomatic decline, can be effected in some patients through the control of comorbidities that would otherwise exacerbate dementia symptoms. In this regard, the number of possible interventions remains as diverse as the number of potential comorbidities. Failure to control seemingly unrelated problems such as congestive heart failure, emphysema, or diabetes mellitus, for example, may exacerbate cognitive and functional impairment, and this increment of secondarily imposed decline may be reversible with better management of these comorbidities. AD (like all degenerative diseases) has an expected rate and pattern of clinical progression. If the pattern or rate of decline strays from what was expected, other contributory factors should be considered and sought.

In vignette A, our asymptomatic 46-year-old engineer wants to prevent or delay the onset of AD. He should be told that nothing has been proven to do that, but in general, healthy lifestyle choices have some supporting data and certainly make sense for his cardiovascular health as well. These include aerobic fitness and exercise, a Mediterranean diet (or similar low-fat, high-vegetable diet), and staying mentally active. As an employed engineer, he probably needs no further mental stimulation, but stress management and mental hygiene are also generally beneficial independent of any role they may play in dementia prevention.

As for his mother, in vignette B, her comorbidities should be monitored and if needed addressed, including her hypothyroidism and blood sugar. Her recent history of beast cancer is also concerning, given the greater-than-expected decline that has occurred since her previous evaluation a year earlier, and further evaluation into the possibility of cancer recurrence should also be considered. Addressing such issues can result in improved patient performance even in the absence of any direct effect on the neurobiology of AD itself.

References

1. Carpenter BD, Strauss ME, Patterson MB. Sleep disturbances in community-dwelling patients with Alzheimer's disease. Clin Gerontol 1995;16:35–49.

2. McCurry SM, Logsdon RG, Teri L, et al. Characteristics of sleep disturbance in community-dwelling Alzheimer's disease patients. J Geriatr Psychaitry Neurol 1999;12:53–59.

3. Hope T, Keene J, Gedling K, et al. Predictors of institutionalization for people with dementia living at home with a carer. Int J Geriatr Psychiatry 1998;13:682–690.

4. McCurry SM, Gibbons LE, Logsdon RG, et al. Nighttime insomnia treatment and education for Alzheimer's disease: a randomized, controlled trial. J Am Geriatr Soc 2005;53:793–802.

5. Shelton PS, Hocking LB. Zolpidem for dementia-related insomnia and nighttime wandering. Ann Pharmacother 1997;31:319–322.

6. Agostini JV, Leo-Summers LS, Inouye SK. Cognitive and other adverse effects of diphenhydramine use in hospitalized older patients. Arch Intern Med 2001;161:2091–2097.

7. Basu R, Dodge H, Stoehr GP, et al. Sedative-hypnotic use of diphenhydramine in a rural, older adult, community-based cohort: effects on cognition. Am J Geriatr Psychiatry 2003;11:205–213.

8. Boeve BF, Silber MH, Ferman TJ, et al. Association of REM sleep behavior disorder and neurodegenerative disease may reflect an underlying synucleinopathy. Mov Disord 2001;16:622–630.

9. Gagnon JF, Postuma RB, Montplaisir J. Update on the pharmacology of REM sleep behavior disorder. Neurology 2006;67:742–747.

10. Caselli RJ. Obstructive sleep apnea, apolipoprotein E e4, and mild cognitive impairment. Sleep Med 2008;9:816–817.

11. Kadotani H, Kadotani T, Young T, et al. Association between apolipoprotein E epsilon4 and sleep-disordered breathing in adults. JAMA 2001;285:2888–2890.

12. Gottlieb DJ, DeStefano AL, Foley DJ, et al. APOE epsilon4 is associated with obstructive sleep apnea/hypopnea: the Sleep Heart Health Study. Neurology 2004;63:664–668.

13. Schor JD, Levkoff SE, Lipsitz LA, et al. Risk factors for delirium in hospitalized elderly. JAMA 1992;267:827–831.

14. Elie M, Cole MG, Primeau FJ, et al. Delirium risk factors in elderly hospitalized patients. J Gen Intern Med 1998;13:204–212.

15. Pisani MA, Murphy TE, Van Ness PH, et al. Characteristics associated with delirium in older patients in a medical intensive care unit. Arch Intern Med 2007;167:1629–1634.

16. Rudolph JL, Jones RN, Levkoff SE, et al. Derivation of a preoperative prediction rule for delirium after cardiac surgery. Circulation 2009;119:229–236.

17. Francis J, Martin D, Kapoor WN. A prospective study of delirium in hospitalized elderly. JAMA 1990;263:1097–1101.

18. Kiely DK, Marcantonio ER, Inouye SK, et al. Persistent delirium predicts greater mortality. J Am Geriatr Soc 2009;57:55–61.

19. McAvay GJ, Van Ness PH, Bogardus ST Jr, et al. Older adults discharged from hospital with delirium: 1-year outcomes. J Am Geriatr Soc 2006;54:1245–1250.

20. Leslie DL, Marcantonio ER, Zhang Y, et al. One-year health care costs associated with delirium in the elderly population. Arch Intern Med 2008;168:27–32.

21. Inouye SK. Delirium in older persons. N Engl J Med 2006;354:1157–1165.

22. Temporal Orientation Test. In Benton AI, Sivan AB, Hamsher K deS, et al. Contributions to Neuropsychological Assessment. A Clinical Manual, 2nd ed. New York: Oxford University Press, 1994.

23. Inouye SK, van Dyck CH, Alessi CA, et al. Clarifying confusion: the confusion assessment method. A new method for detection of delirium. Ann Intern Med 1990;113:941–948.

24. Marcantonio ER, Flacker JM, Wright JR, et al. Reducing delirium after hip fracture. J Am Geriatr Soc 2001;49:516–522.

25. Kalisvaart KJ, de Jonghe JF, Bogaards MJ, et al. Haloperidol prophylaxis for elderly hip surgery patients at risk for delirium: a randomized placebo-controlled study. J Am Geriatr Soc 2005;53:1658–1666.

26. Prakanrattana UU. Efficacy of risperidone for prevention of postoperative delirium in cardiac surgery. Anesth Intensive Care 2007;35:714–719.

27. Petersen RC, Thomas RG, Grundman M, et al. Vitamin E and donepezil for the treatment of mild cognitive impairment. N Engl J Med 2005;352:2379–2388.

28. Aisen PS, Schneider LS, Sano M, et al. High-dose B vitamin supplementation and cognitive decline in Alzheimer disease: a randomized controlled trial. JAMA 2008;300:1774–1783.

29. Aisen PS, Schafer KA, Grundman M, et al. Effects of rofecoxib or naproxen vs placebo on Alzheimer disease progression: a randomized controlled trial. JAMA 2003;289:2819–2826.

30. Shumaker SA, Legault C, Thal, L, et al. Estrogen plus progestin and the incidence of dementia and mild cognitive impairment in postmenopausal women: the Women's Health Initiative Memory Study, a randomized controlled trial. JAMA 2003;289:2651–2662.

31. DeKosky ST, Williamson JD, Fitzpatrick AL, et al. Gingko biloba for prevention of dementia: a randomized controlled trial. JAMA 2008;300:2253–2262.

32. Etnier JL, Caselli RJ, Reiman EM, et al. Cognitive performance in older women relative to ApoE-e4 genotype and aerobic fitness. Med Sci Sports Exerc 2007;39:199–207.

33. Laurin D, Verreault R, Lindsay J, et al. Physical activity and risk of cognitive impairment and dementia in elderly persons. Arch Neurol 2001;58:498–504.

34. Ravaglia G, Forti P, Lucicesare A, et al. Physical activity and dementia risk in the elderly: findings from a prospective Italian study. Neurology 2008;70:1786–1794.

35. Larson EB, Wang L, Bowen JD, et al. Exercise is associated with reduced risk for incident dementia among persons 65 years of age and older. Ann Intern Med 2006;144:73–81.

36. Burns JM, Cronk BB, Anderson HS, et al. Cardiorespiratory fitness and brain atrophy in early Alzheimer disease. Neurology 2008;71:210–216.

37. Lautenschlager NT, Cox KL, Flicker L, et al. Effect of physical activity on cognitive function in older adults at risk for Alzheimer disease. JAMA 2008;300:1027–1037.

38. Wilson RS, Mendes De Leon CF, Barnes LL, et al. Participation in cognitively stimulating activities and risk of incident Alzheimer's disease. JAMA 2002;287:742–748.

39. Scarmeas N, Levy G, Tang MX, et al. Influence of leisure activity on the incidence of Alzheimer's disease. Neurology 2001;57:2236–2242.

40. Valenzuela M, Sachdev P. Can cognitive exercise prevent the onset of dementia? Systematic review of randomized clinical trials with longitudinal followup. Am J Geriatr Psychiatry 2009;17:179–187.

41. Scarmeas N, Stern Y, Tang MX, et al. Mediterranean diet and risk for Alzheimer's disease. Ann Neurol 2006;59:912–921.

42. Perez-Jimenez F, Alvarez de Cienfuegos G, Badimon L, et al. International conference on the healthy effect of virgin olive oil. Eur J Clin Invest 2005;35:421–424.

43. Ruitenberg A, van Swieten JC, Witteman JC, et al. Alcohol consumption and risk of dementia: the Rotterdam Study. Lancet 2002;359:281–286.

44. Ringman JM, Frautschy SA, Cole GM, et al. A potential role of the curry spice curcumin in Alzheimer's disease. Curr Alzheimer Res 2005;2:131–136.

45. Zandi PP, Anthony JC, Khachaturian AS, et al. Reduced risk of Alzheimer disease in users of antioxidant vitamin supplements: the Cache County Study. Arch Neurol 2004;61:82–88.

46. Commenges D, Scotet V, Renaud S, et al. Intake of flavonoids and risk of dementia. Eur J Epidemiol 2000;16:357–363.

47. Engelhart MJ, Geerlings MI, Ruitenberg A, et al. Dietary intake of antioxidants and risk of Alzheimer disease. JAMA 2002;287:3223–3229.

48. Kalmijn S, Feskens EJ, Launer LJ, et al. Polyunsaturated fatty acids, antioxidants, and cognitive function in very old men. Am J Epidemiol 1997;145:33–41.

49. Luchsinger JA, Tang MX, Shea S, et al. Caloric intake and the risk of Alzheimer disease. Arch Neurol 2002;59:1258–1263.

50. Haag MD, Hofman A, Koudstaal PJ, et al. Statins are associated with a reduced risk of Alzheimer disease regardless of lipophilicity. The Rotterdam Study. J Neurol Neurosurg Psychiatry 2009;80:13–17.

51. Arvanitakis Z, Schneider JA, Wilson RS, et al. Statins, incident Alzheimer disease, change in cognitive function, and neuropathology. Neurology 2008; 70:1795–1802.

52. Sparks DL, Connor DJ, Sabbagh MN, et al. Circulating cholesterol levels, apolipoprotein E genotype and dementia severity influence the benefit of atorvastatin treatment of Alzheimer's disease: results of the Alzheimer's Disease Cholesterol Lowering Treatment (ADCLT) trial. Acta Neurol Scand Suppl 2006;185:3–7.

53. Winblad B, Jelic V, Kershaw P, et al. Effects of statins on cognitive function in patients with Alzheimer's disease in galantamine clinical trials. Drugs Aging 2007;24:57–61.

54. DeFelice FG, Vieira MN, Bomfim TR, et al. Protection of synapses against Alzheimer's-linked toxins: insulin signalling prevents the pathogenic binding of abeta oligomers. Proc Natl Acad Sci USA 2009;106:1971–1976.

55. Moloney AM, Griffin RJ, Timmons S, et al. Defects in IGF-1 receptor, insulin receptor, and IRS-1/2 in Alzheimer's disease indicate possible resistance to IGF-1 and insulin signaling. Neurobiol Aging May 12 2008 [Epub].

56. Strum JC, Shehee R, Virley D, et al. Rosiglitazone induces mitochondrial biogenesis in mouse brain. J Alzheimers Dis 2007;11:45–51.

57. Ronnemaa E, Zethelius B, Sundelof J, et al. Impaired insulin secretion increases the risk of Alzheimer's disease. Neurology 2008;71:1065–1071.

58. Muller M, Tang MX, Scupf N, et al. Metabolic syndrome and dementia risk in a multiethnic elderly cohort. Dementia Geriatr Cogn Disord 2007;24:185–192.

59. Risner ME, Saunders AM, Altman JF, et al. Efficacy of rosiglitazone in a genetically defined population with mild-to-moderate Alzheimer's disease. Pharmacogenomics J 2006;6:222–224.

60. Roses AD, Saunders AM, Huang Y, et al. Complex disease-associated pharmacogenetics: drug efficacy, drug safety, and confirmation of a pathogenetic hypothesis (Alzheimer's disease). Pharmacogenomics J 2007;7:10–28.

Section D

Nonpharmacological management

Unfortunately, there are important lifestyle issues that require attention because pharmacotherapy falls well short of symptomatic reversal. Table D.1 summarizes some of these, and they are described in more detail in the following chapters.

Table D.1 Nonpharmacological Interventions	
	Action
Driving	MCI: caution, q 6 month rechecks
	Mild (and worse) Alzheimer's disease: stop completely
Weapons	Secure, unload
Finances	MCI: caution, observe
	Mild (and worse) Alzheimer's Disease: stop completely
Advance directive	Power of attorney
	Legal guardianship
	Medical directives and living will
Assisted living	If available, capable, and willing caregiver, placement only as needed.
	If none, consider assisted living with MCI (and worse).
	If not capable of dressing, feeding, toileting independently, consider skilled nursing facility.

Chapter 12

Acute interventions

Driving

One of the more difficult lifestyle changes for patients with dementia to accept is not driving. According to the Practice Parameter of the Quality Standards Subcommittee of the American Academy of Neurology (1), patients with MCI should be cautioned, and rechecked every 6 months, but if felt to be safe, may continue to drive. Some forms of MCI, however, that primarily affect visuospatial or executive skills may preclude safe driving despite the practice parameter, and such patients should not drive (2). Patients who have progressed past the MCI stage and are considered to have mild-stage dementia should not drive at all (1).

Physicians should be aware of reporting requirements in their area. California, Oregon, and Pennsylvania require physicians to report the diagnosis of dementia, and California and Pennsylvania hold physicians liable for motor vehicle accidents if they fail to report such patients. Several states even have mandatory relicensing procedures that involve some form of medical assessment that is based on age (3).

There are many reasons why patients with dementia should not drive. Patients with visual variant AD have disabling visual impairment (4). Patients with apraxic variant AD have severe motor impairment, and most also have visual impairment. Patients with aphasic variant AD might appear to have the motor skills for driving, but due to the speech disturbance occurring within the context of a dementing degenerative brain disease would be ill equipped to explain themselves in the event of a mishap, and legally would be difficult to defend if challenged. Impaired attention, inability to multitask, and other cognitive disturbances in addition to memory loss all impair driving skills, as shown on actual road tests (5–8) as well as on driving simulation tests (9–12). These impairments result in a two- to eightfold increase in the rate of collisions in AD patients who continue driving (1).

Simply telling a patient with dementia not to drive often is not sufficient, and many continue to drive even after they develop evident driving impairment despite admonitions not to drive (5,6). Patients may take a driving test, and

Table 12.1 Driving Laws Related To Alzheimer's Disease

	Mandatory Reporting, Cognitive Impairment	Mandatory Reporting, Other Diagnosis	Physician Report Immune from Legal Action by Patients	Physician Liable for MVA if Nonreport	Age-Based Required Evaluation
Alabama	no	no	yes	?	no
Alaska	no	no	no	?	no
Arizona	no	no	yes	?	no
Arkansas	no	no	no	?	no
California	Alzheimer's, related	epilepsy, etc.	yes for required	yes	no
Colorado	no	no	yes	?	no
Connecticut	no	no	no	?	no
Delaware	no	LOC	yes	no	no
D.C.	no	no	no	?	yes, 70
Florida	no	no	yes	?	no
Georgia	no	no	yes	?	no
Hawaii	no	no	no	?	no
Idaho	no	no	no	?	no
Illinois	no	no	yes	?	yes, 75
Indiana	no	no	no	?	no
Iowa	no	no	yes	?	no
Kansas	no	no	yes	?	no
Kentucky	no	no	yes	?	no
Louisiana	no	no	yes	?	no
Maine	no	no	yes	?	no
Maryland	no	no	yes	?	no
Massachusetts	no	no	no	?	no
Michigan	no	no	no	?	no
Minnesota	no	no	yes	?	no
Mississippi	no	no	no	?	no
Missouri	no	no	yes	?	no
Montana	no	no	yes	?	no
Nebraska	no	no	no	?	no
Nevada	no	epilepsy	no	yes	no

Table 12.1 *Continued*

	Mandatory Reporting, Cognitive Impairment	Mandatory Reporting, Other Diagnosis	Physician Report Immune from Legal Action by Patients	Physician Liable for MVA if Nonreport	Age-Based Required Evaluation
New Hampshire	no	no	no	?	yes, 75
New Jersey	no	recurrent LOC	recurrent LOC	no	no
New Mexico	no	no	yes	?	no
New York	no	no	no	?	no
North Carolina	no	no	yes	?	no
North Dakota	no	no	yes	?	no
Ohio	no	no	no	?	no
Oklahoma	no	no	yes	?	no
Oregon	cognitive/ functional	LOC	yes	no	50 (eye)
Pennsylvania	any impairs driving	any	yes	yes	45 (physical/ eye)
Rhode Island	no	no	yes	?	no
South Carolina	no	no	no	?	no
South Dakota	no	no	no	?	no
Tennessee	no	no	no	?	no
Texas	no	no	yes	?	no
Utah	no	no	yes	?	no
Vermont	no	no	no	?	no
Virginia	no	no	yes	?	no
Washington	no	no	no	?	no
West Virginia	no	no	no	?	no
Wisconsin	No	no	yes	?	no
Wyoming	No	no	yes	?	no

LOC, loss of consciousness; MVA, motor vehicle accident.

Adapted from Summary of Medical Advisory Board Practices in the U.S., June 18, 2003. National Highway Transportation and Safety Administration/Transanalytics LLC.

when they do, 40% to 60% fail (13,14), but losing their license only makes it illegal for them to drive. The most effective way to stop a patient from driving is to remove his or her access to car keys or the car itself. This is not always easy to accomplish and has caused some patients to become belligerent, so care must be used in managing this very difficult but critical issue.

Weapons and Other Safety Issues

Relatively little has been written about proper handling of weapons in "dementia households" (15), save that the issue exists and would seem to pose a serious risk. One study found that gun ownership was prevalent in 60% of these households, and that the guns were known to be deliberately kept unloaded in only 17% of them. Common sense would argue that weapons should be addressed at least as consistently as driving, and perhaps with even greater sensitivity. Secured storage sites, unloading the weapons, and similar measures should be undertaken.

Regarding other aspects of home safety, the home environment should remain familiar—that is, rearranging furniture or redesigning the interior is ill advised in the context of dementia. Rooms should have uncluttered floors and walls with ample lighting, including a nightlight to prevent falls and injuries. Occasionally, photographs of family members and friends can lead to confusion regarding who is in the home; if this occurs, such pictures should be removed. Other examples of home modifications include installing locks on cabinets, cupboards, and ovens and removing knobs on the stove. Poisonous or harmful substances and sharp objects should be secured out of reach. Caregivers should be encouraged to register patients in the Alzheimer's Association's Safe Return Program, an identification program for dementia patients who have a tendency to wander (www.alz.org).

Protecting Finances

Patients with dementia are at risk for mishandling money. This can manifest as difficulty making change; misplacing wallets, credit cards, and checkbooks; inability to manage household finances and bank accounts; poor investment judgment; and frank victimization by scam artists. Additionally, patients with executive variant AD may develop hording behavior and spend extraordinary amounts of money on multiple copies of the same item, such as magazine subscriptions. The consequences of such errors can range from a minor nuisance to financial ruin. It is therefore essential that a reliable and responsible individual assume control of finances. If this cannot be readily achieved by a trusted family member, then legal recourse should be sought to secure the patient's estate and create a vehicle that will provide for his or her necessary care.

References

1. Dubinsky RM, Stein AC, Lyons K. Risk of driving and Alzheimer's disease (an evidence-based review): report of the Quality Standards Subcommittee of the American Academy of Neurology. Neurology 2000;54:2205–2211.

2. Dawson JD, Anderson SW, Uc EY, et al. Predictors of driving safety in early Alzheimer's disease. Neurology 2009;72:521–527.

3. Summary of Medical Advisory Board Practices in the U.S., June 18, 2003. National Highway Transportation and Safety Administration/Transanalytics LLC.

4. Caselli RJ. Visual syndromes as the presenting feature of degenerative brain disease. Sem Neurol 2000;20:139–144.

5. Drachman DA, Swearer JM. Driving and Alzheimer's disease: the risk of crashes. Neurology 1993;43:2448–2456.

6. Logsdon RG, Teri L, Larson EB. Driving and Alzheimer's disease. J Gen Intern Med 1992;7:583–588.

7. Fitten LJ, Perryman KM, Wilkinson CJ, et al. Alzheimer and vascular dementias and driving. JAMA 1995;273:1360–1365.

8. Hunt LA, Murphy CF, Carr D, et al. Reliability of the Washington University Road Test: a performance-based assessment for drivers with dementia of the Alzheimer type. Arch Neurol 1997;54:707–712.

9. Duchek JM, Hunt L, Ball K, et al. Attention and driving performance in Alzheimer's disease. J Gerontol 1998;53:P130–P141.

10. Rebok GW, Keyl PM, Bylsma FW, et al. The effects of Alzheimer's disease on driving-related abilities. Alz Dis Rel Disord 1994;8:228–240.

11. Rizzo M, Reinach S, McGehee D, et al. Simulated car crashes and crash predictors in Alzheimer disease. Arch Neurol 1997;54:545–551.

12. Cox DJ, McQuillian WC, Thorndike FP, et al. Evaluating driving performance of outpatients with Alzheimer's disease. J Am Board Fam Prac 1998;11:264–271.

13. Hunt L, Morris JC, Edwards D, et al. Driving performance in persons with mild senile dementia. J Am Geriatr Soc 1993;41:747–752.

14. Fox GK, Bowden SC, Bashford GM, et al. Alzheimer disease and driving: prediction and assessment of driving performance. J Am Geriatr Soc 1997;45:949–953.

14. Mendez MF. Dementia and guns. J Am Geriatr Soc 1996;44:409–410.

15. Spangenberg KB, Wagner MT, Hendrix S, Bachman DL. Firearm presence in households of patients with Alzheimer's disease and related dementias. J Am Geriatr Soc 1996;47:1183–1186.

Chapter 13

Communicating with dementia patients

AD impairs the patient's language and ability to communicate. The severity of language impairment varies between patients, but language impairment generally follows a trajectory that parallels cognitive and functional decline. Coupled with reduced perceptual and attentional skills that impede the patient's ability to handle competing stimuli and filter out environmental noise, patients lose their coping skills and become increasingly isolated from the world and others around them (1). As verbal comprehension worsens, patients become increasingly dependent on nonverbal communication, including body language, intonation, and gesture. Problems with communication often result in "acting out" behaviors. It may be difficult for a caregiver to be certain about what is causing a patient's pleasure or displeasure in his or her reactions to an event or to the caregiver (2), but responses are more likely to be positive (and not "acting out") when patients perceive the caregiver's speech to be respectful, caring, not controlling, and conveying a sense of the patient's own competence (3). There are even some specialized training programs for communication skills in caregivers (2–6).

In addition to focusing on caregiver communication, some programs have focused on the patient:

- A Memory Club for people with early-stage dementia and their caregivers to provide information and support and to discuss AD issues. The program has been "rated positively" by participants (7).

- A program using storytelling to encourage people with dementia to take part in associated conversations, helping them to remember and talk of past experiences. Increases in spontaneous conversation and group interactions were noted (8).

- A program designed to help elders with early-stage dementia and their caregivers participate in five aspects of decision making: information received; being listened to; expressing an opinion; time allowed for reflection on the decisions; and the possibility of changing their mind (9).

Suggested Communication Strategies

While there are few evidence-based communication interventions, there is broad agreement on best practices. The following suggestions for successful communication with AD patients are based upon the literature as well as our own experience and can be helpful for clinicians, families, and caregivers:

1. Listen carefully and fully to what the patient says. Examine what seems like incoherent speech for themes or key words. Repeat them back to the patient and observe the response. Often families can "tap into" meaning with careful listening.
2. Pay careful attention to the patient's body language to determine the emotional importance of the communication.
3. Approach the person with respect. Avoid "talking down" to him or her or using childlike voice tones.
4. Always assume the patient understands what is being said.
5. Talk to the patient and the caregiver. Do not inadvertently ignore the patient when discussing his or her condition.
6. Avoid complicated explanations; avoid trying to reason with the patient.
7. Discuss the illness with the person, reinforcing that AD is "just an illness."
8. Ask "yes" and "no" questions.
9. Touching a hand may enhance attention as well demonstrate that you care.
10. Gently leading/cueing the patient through the (verbal) request may be helpful.
11. Showing and touching physical objects and/or pictures may help with memory and assist with conversation.
12. Exercise forgiveness and don't correct mistakes.
13. To diffuse tense situations, agree with the person, apologize that he or she is upset, and plead ignorance.
14. Reminiscing about positive past life events may be a good way to decrease anxiety (10). The technique involves helping the patient communicate by tapping into long-established memories. Reminiscence often helps to calm the patient and promote feelings of well-being. Reminiscence can also help the listener to organize the patient's language into a more coherent concept (11,12). (However, this is a not universally appropriate technique. Obsessive reminiscence and rumination occurs when the patient becomes "stuck" on certain memories, causing disruption of the environmental milieu and interpersonal relationships that can alienate caregivers and significant others. Obsessive reminiscing can be an indication of delirium, anxiety, depression, or perseveration.)
15. Always begin communication by eliminating any possible background distractions, such as the TV, radio, or too many people talking at once.
16. Make sure glasses, hearing aids (with batteries), and dentures are all in place.

17. Allow ample time for the person to communicate. Try not to finish his or her sentences.

18. Remain still and with the person while you are talking. This will make it easier to follow the conversation and demonstrates a sincere, empathetic approach.

19. When the person has difficulty finding a word, consider asking him or her to explain in a different way, or try giving clues. You may also try to guess the meaning and ask if you are correct.

20. Ask the person to show you what he or she is referring to. Pointing to an object may also help get the message across.

21. Try to avoid allowing your own stress and exasperation to show, as it will increase tension.

22. Incorporating information in your conversation that tells the patient where he or she is, what is happening around him or her, and whom he or she is with, and using descriptors with names, can enhance security and orientation (13).

23. For patients with severe language impairment, be aware that certain words are very high impact and may be understood to the exclusion of all else, including proper context.

24. Some patients retain a defensive attitude of denial about their diagnosis or become very depressed at the words, "Alzheimer's disease." Softer terms that will be understood by the family, such as "memory loss," may help to avoid aggravating such a patient.

References

1. Hall G, Buckwalter K. A conceptual model for planning and evaluating care of the client with Alzheimer's disease. Arch Psychiatric Nurs 1987;1(6):399–406.

2. Polk D. Communication and family caregiving for Alzheimer's dementia: Linking attributions and problematic integration. Health Communication 2005;18(3):257–273.

3. Small J, Perry J, Lewis J. Perceptions of family caregivers' psychosocial behavior when communicating with spouses who have Alzheimer's disease. Am J Alzheimers Dis Other Dementias 2005;20(5):281–289.

4. Acton G. Developing prescriptions to increase collaborative social communications in persons with dementia. South Online J Nurs Res 2008;8:2. Accessed January 20, 2009; available at: http://snrs.org/publications/SOJNR_articles2/Vol08Num02A.html#Acton

5. Back A, Arnold R. Dealing with conflict in caring for the seriously ill: "it was just out of the question." JAMA 2005;293(11):1374–1381.

6. de la Cuesta C. The craft of care: family care of relatives with advanced dementia. Qualitative Health Res 2005;15(7):881–896.

7. Zarit S, Femia E, Watson J, et al. Memory Club: A group intervention for people with early-stage dementia and their care partners. Gerontologist 2004;44(2):262–269.

8. Holm A, Lepp M, Ringsberg K. Dementia: Involving patients in storytelling—a caring intervention. A pilot study. J Clin Nurs 2005;14(2):256–263.

9. Tyrrell J, Genin N, Myslinski M. Freedom of choice and decision-making in health and social care: Views of older patients with early-stage dementia and their carers. Dementia 2006;5(4):479–502.

10. Puentes WJ. Simple reminiscence: A stress-adaptation model of the phenomenon. Issues Mental Health Nurs 2002;23:497–511.

11. Puentes WJ. Using an associated trends framework to understand the meaning of obsessive reminiscence. J Gerontol Nurs 2008;34(7):44–49.

12. Sabat SR. The Experience of Alzheimer's Disease: Life Through a Tangled Veil. Malden, MA: Blackwell, 2001.

13. Hall G. Communication Skills in Alzheimer's Disease. MAPS Modules, no. 10. Phoenix: Family & Community Services Program, Banner Alzheimer's Institute, 2008.

Chapter 14

Managing problem behaviors, aggression, and violence

AD may be known to the lay public as a disorder that is characterized by intellectual impairment such as memory loss, but to caregivers, both lay and professional, the most challenging aspects of the disease are its behavioral disturbances. These can range in severity from relatively minor nuisances such as arranging clothes to frankly dangerous behavior that can include physical violence. The severity of the behavioral disturbance does not follow a simple parallel with the severity of intellectual impairment, although in general the likelihood of any behavioral disturbance increases with dementia severity. Behavior also tends to deteriorate during the late afternoon and early evening, a phenomenon called "sundowning." It may reflect a variety of factors such as fatigue, lower light intensity (impairing vision), and diurnal endocrinological changes, as well as other factors. Ultimately, any behavior that a caregiver identifies as problematic, especially if it interferes with effective caregiving or caregiver health, should be addressed (1).

A qualitative study reported that caregivers who had not received specific training on dementia care used "ignoring," "walking away," and "accepting behavior" 52% of the time to manage behaviors. This resulted in significantly more episodes of refusing care, repetitive behaviors, incontinent episodes, sundown syndrome, night wakening, and psychosis (2). Another study demonstrated the critical issue of caregiver's discussing the illness with the patient. Caregivers who did not discuss the disease with their patient distanced themselves, causing increases in the frequency of behavior problems, including activity disturbances, paranoia, and anxiety. These behaviors in turn led to increased closeout of the patient by the caregiver, further worsening behaviors (3).

Use of nonpharmacological measures, including services and environmental management, can often reduce or eliminate the need for medications (2). For example, physicians report that 71% of behavior problems reported in nursing homes involve refusal of personal care (4), for which medications provide little benefit. Ideally, a goal should be to minimize the use of psychotropic medications, and to that end nonpharmacological interventions can be considered in almost all but the most dangerous types of situations.

Common Behavioral Changes in Dementia Patients

Challenging behaviors can and do occur at all stages of disease severity. Here are some common examples.

Early Dementia

- Demanding to leave during an activity or event, even if it had been anticipated with excitement
- Seeming selfish or rude
- Accusing family members of stealing items the person has hidden, or blaming "outsiders" for taking things
- Hiding things
- Telling stories that are known not to be true (confabulation)
- Insisting on driving or doing other things that threaten safety despite obvious limitations
- Having sudden mood changes
- Increased interest in sexual activity
- Repetitive questioning

Moderate Dementia

- Waking up in the middle of the night to get dressed and start the day
- Not recognizing familiar settings, home, or family members late in the afternoon
- Threatening family members with physical violence
- Demanding to go home when already at home
- Becoming confused, irritated, or belligerent late in the day
- Refusing to bathe, go to the doctor, or go on social outings for no apparent reason
- Walking away from home or getting lost
- Pacing back and forth without stopping
- Thinking there are extra people or children in the home
- Perseverative masturbation
- Vegetative behaviors

Advanced Dementia

- Asking for the caregiver when the caregiver is in the room
- Thinking television, mirrors, and family pictures are extra silent people in the room
- Having spontaneous or repetitive loud vocalizations
- Day/night sleep–wake reversal
- REM sleep disorder
- Return of primitive grasp reflex and mistaking this for "grabbing"

More serious behavioral disturbances, including aggression and violence, will be considered separately later in this chapter.

Categories of Factors That Can Trigger Behavioral Alterations

When confronted with a report of a behavioral problem, the physician must try to determine the triggers and potential consequences of the behavior. Unexpected changes in behavior are often triggered by things that can be controlled, such as changes in daily routine. Behavioral effects may lag precipitating triggers by up to 48 hours (although usually they occur more quickly than that). It is important to know how many days each week and the time of day a behavior occurs. Have the caregiver estimate the severity of the behavior as he or she would pain, on a 1-to-10 scale, with 10 being the worst behavior imaginable. Six categories of triggers include:

1. Fatigue. Patients with dementia fatigue early. Routine "time-outs" must be built into a schedule or the patient will become agitated late in the day or will be up at night. Have the caregiver schedule two rest periods during the day to minimize the potential for dementia.

2. Change of routine or location. Changes such as having guests, holiday decorations, and especially relocating to a long-term care facility will cause anxiety and anger. Travel is an especially difficult time.

3. Perceptions of loss. Losing driving or reading skills and becoming unable to participate fully can cause depression. Lost activities must be replaced with new activities and people must talk with the patient about why these changes are taking place, so the disease is the villain and the patient can grieve for his or her losses. Activities are a critical yet often overlooked aspect of dementia care.

4. Overwhelming or misleading sensory input. Noisy places and large groups tend to cause excess disability in people with dementia early in the disease. Patients with moderate to advanced dementia will report television as "children in the house." Seemingly benign things like mirrors and family pictures become extra people. The misperceptions caused by this are not a true psychosis, but rather pseudohallucinations that disappear once the source is removed.

5. Excessive demand. Anxiety and even paranoia can be provoked when people insist that the patient participate in activities that exceed his or her capacity—for example, when family members try to have the patient focus on knowing the date and time.

6. Delirium. This is a medically more serious disturbance that requires formal evaluation and sometimes medical intervention (as discussed in the pharmacotherapy section). Infections (especially urinary tract infections, pneumonia, and cellulitis) may be the most common causes, but pain, medication interactions, and trauma are other common precipitants of delirium (2,5,6).

Finally, in advanced/terminal dementia the patient is unable to communicate. Triggers to be considered in this context include unmet basic needs, such as hunger or pain.

Interventions: General Considerations

There are few if any evidence-based interventions for specific behavioral problems. Despite the family's best efforts, one day the patient begins to scream, doesn't recognize the home, or wanders away. How can the family be counseled when this happens? The following interventions have been developed for direct in-home family caregivers and are considered "best practices" among clinical experts (1,7):

1. Recognize that the problem is temporary and will pass. Make sure family members are safe until it passes.
2. Do not argue with or confront the patient. Consider that he or she may be frightened or panicky. Fear can be magnified inadvertently if the caregiver feels that the patient is not aware of his or her memory loss and confusion, leading the caregiver to avoid discussing the disease and upsetting the person with the disease, thereby worsening anxiety (3). Tell the patient you understand and intend to help.
3. Give the patient something to do, or ask him or her to help you do something.
4. Get the patient to a quiet place where he or she can rest briefly.
5. If it is the middle of the night, offer a snack and get the patient to an easy chair. Do not try to convince the patient that it is night by showing him or her it is dark outside.
6. If the patient does not recognize the home, try driving around the block together or reassuring the patient that this is the place where you will spend the night (implying it is a hotel). Reassure the patient that you will both go home tomorrow.
7. Try calling one of the patient's children to offer reassurance. This sometimes works when all else fails.
8. If the episode does not resolve within an hour or so and is escalating to the point of physical or potential physical aggression, it may be necessary to have a medical evaluation by the physician or nearest urgent care center or emergency room. Do not try to get an agitated confused person into the car; call the paramedics.

Interventions for Specific Nonviolent Problems

Bathing

Patients can go through a phase where they either refuse to bathe or say they have already finished their bath:

- Let the patient choose the time of day to bathe.
- Make sure to have a warm towel and fluffy robe to prevent chilling.
- Sometimes bathing at the sink is sufficient; this can help allay the patient's fear of falling in the tub.
- Towel baths can help the institutionalized person accept bathing.

- Remind him or her of a special occasion for which bathing is needed (e.g., "we can't go out for lunch until you bathe").
- Associate a pleasant experience with the bath (such as a food treat or music).
- Make sure to check the temperature of the bathwater or shower to prevent freezing or scalding.
- Color the bathwater or use bubble bath.
- Make sure there is a nonskid mat or surface in the tub.
- Try a hand-held showerhead so water does not hit the patient's head.
- Allow the person to bathe with underwear on.
- Sing during bath time to relieve the tension or have some soft music in the background.
- Compliment the person after the bath.
- Sometimes a bath aide can do what the caregiver is unable to.

Wearing the Same Clothing Day After Day

This is an indication that the patient cannot handle change and is normal for people with memory loss. Try purchasing several identical outfits when shopping. Then, when the person takes one set of dirty clothing off, remove it and replace it with an identical set of clean clothing.

Hiding Things

Hiding things often represents a concern about theft.

- Remove valuables from the house whenever possible. Remember, these possessions still belong to the person and cannot legally be dispersed using the person's will. Take larger valuables such as the family crystal, silverware, and china, and pack them away. Label the cartons "books" or something that does not attract attention and place them in a safe area.
- Place jewelry not used daily in a safety deposit box.
- Take jewelry worn daily and have it appraised. Have the jeweler remove the most valuable stones and place them in a safety deposit box. Replace the valuable stones with inexpensive material such as cubic zirconium and return to the patient. Jewelry sent to the nursing home or assisted living facility is likely to disappear.
- Put "clappers" on house and car keys so they beep when lost; have a routine place, like a basket at the door, and remind the patient to drop keys or other essential items (wallet, glasses) in it when entering the home.
- Some of the more common hiding places are under the mattress, in books, in the hems of curtains, under the paper in back of pictures or mirrors, under pillows, in food containers, in the freezer, behind bricks in the basement, in breakfront cabinets, wadded in tissues in toilet paper cardboard cylinders, or in the trash.
- Make duplicates of keys and other items. (However, losing the car keys is a way to have a loved one stop driving. This is one example where family can decide to let the keys "stay lost" and not volunteer another set.)

Refusing Adult Day Programs and In-Home Care

Many patients refuse to go to adult day programs or to allow in-home respite services.

- Have the caregiver stay with the person in day care for 2 or 3 days until the patient becomes familiar with the staff and routine. If he or she feels uneasy about the day care setting or upset about being put in a place with people more impaired than he or she is, perhaps another family member might help out. Research shows that people who attend adult day programming stay at home longer and adapt better to new circumstances, especially placement.
- Have extra help in the home as early as possible in the course of the disease so the person is used to having others around. A cleaning person is a good starting place. Make sure that family members participate in care on a regular basis; if possible, friends should take the patient out whenever possible.
- Often the patient becomes enraged when a service provider or family member is used for respite. The caregiver should stress to the patient that a break for time alone is needed and should gently reinforce that staying alone or going along is not an option. The caregiver should emphasize that efforts will be made to find respite workers who the patient likes. As the patient becomes accustomed to the day program or respite worker, his or her anger will subside. Successful adaptation to respite will keep the patient at home longer and will help preserve the well-being of the caregiver.

Made-up Stories

AD causes memory loss, and patients tend to "fill in the blanks" when trying to recall an event. Caregivers should understand that as a rule anything the patient says is fine as long as safety is not compromised. They do not need to, and probably should not, correct that patient. If necessary (for the caregiver's stress level), changing the subject is a safer strategy.

Repeated Questions

When the patient asks a question over and over, most often it has to do with when or where something will happen.

- Avoid announcing plans more than 24 hours in advance because it can precipitate obsessive questions.
- Sometimes a question is asked more than once because of a different underlying concern. For example, a patient repeatedly asking what day it is may actually be concerned that he or she will miss, for example, church. Identifying why the patient is asking can sometimes help the caregiver reassure him or her that "you won't miss church" (although the patient may forget this response too).

Wandering, Pacing, and Eloping

- Wandering involves repeatedly walking, almost aimlessly, often getting into things and rummaging. Most people with dementia will wander at some point during the disease. While it is annoying, it is generally harmless unless the person attempts to leave or falls. It is important to put things away that might become broken and remove anything that might cause the person to trip, such as throw rugs or exposed electrical cords. One good approach is to redirect the patient to activities such as music, crafts, helping you cook, or a busy box. People who pace and/or wander tend to do well in adult day programming.

- Pacing is continuous walking back and forth, usually at a brisk pace. People who pace may not stop to eat or participate in activities. Wandering and pacing raise the risk of elopement. Recommend that the family secure doors when unattended and use Home Safe Bracelets from the Alzheimer's Association. Another option is to strategically locate a recliner near an object of visual interest in the pacing loop, such as a bird feeder, which will encourage the person to stop and rest.

- Eloping refers to leaving a specific area without the knowledge and approval of the caregiver. Caregivers must consider their loved ones at risk even though they have never left home before. Some precautions include keeping doors and windows locked when not in use and placing slide bolts at the bottom of exterior and basement doors. The slide bolts need to be easy to open, yet few people with dementia look down to find them.

Hallucinations

Visual hallucinations are rare in "uncomplicated" AD but are a typical accompaniment of dementia with Lewy bodies. They also can occur within the context of an acute delirium superimposed on the underlying dementia. Treatment of hallucinations is primarily medical. However, three phenomena are commonly mistaken for hallucinations. First, they should not be confused with misperceptions of true environmental stimuli. Patients who look at mirrors or photographs and believe them to be silent people are better treated by removing the mirrors and pictures. Second, patients with Capgras syndrome (reduplicative paramnesia) fail to sense the familiarity associated with previously known people and places and accuse caregivers of being "the other" person, or their home as not their home. This is a consequence of dementia progression and does not respond well to medication. Third, vivid dreams and dream enactment behavior are common in the synucleinopathies that include dementia with Lewy bodies, Parkinson's disease, and multiple system atrophy and is caused by REM sleep behavior disorder. Discontinuing potentially aggravating medications sometimes is all that is needed. It is otherwise treated only when necessary, usually with low-dose clonazepam at bedtime.

Aggression and Violence

Preventing aggressive and violent behavior through the previously discussed measures will diminish the chances of a true behavioral emergency. However, even under the best circumstances, violent behavior can still emerge as a reflection of the disease process itself. If the patient is threatening the caregiver verbally or physically, it must be dealt with as an emergency or a potential emergency. Assume the caregiver may be in danger and ask if he or she has an emergency plan in place. If danger seems imminent or violence has already occurred, emergency medical services should be activated (call 911), and hospitalization or institutionalization may be necessary. Such situations usually require pharmacological intervention, and some patients may be able to return home after they have been stabilized and deemed safe.

Verbal Aggression

Verbal aggression should be addressed promptly to prevent the situation from escalating to physical aggression. Some of the more common techniques for diffusing verbal aggression include the following:

- Agree with the patient's statements. You cannot win an argument with a dementia patient who has become verbally aggressive, and disagreeing risks inflaming the situation further.
- Apologize if the patient is blaming you or others for something such as restricted driving or the misfortune of the disease itself, since it is more difficult to argue with someone who is sympathetic. However, if the patient is accusing you of a crime for which, if proven guilty, you would deserve punishment, such as theft or infidelity (two very common themes of paranoid delusions), it becomes a fine line to walk between trying to be agreeable and acknowledging how painful that must feel versus seeming to confirm the patient's paranoid delusion (with its potential repercussions). Medications are more useful in this circumstance, when available.
- Say you don't know what the patient is referring to. For example, if the car keys have been "lost" in an effort to stop the patient from driving, you may act concerned and offer to help with the search (that should end with eventual distraction to another topic and not with the return of the keys).
- In patients who have difficulty communicating, such as those with a severe aphasic component to their dementia, sudden rage may seem random and the cause impossible to decipher. If acting in a sympathetic fashion fails, sometimes removing yourself from the situation, such as going into another room to "find something," will help. This time away may help to de-escalate the situation.

Physical Aggression

When violence occurs, caregivers often report mixed feelings of disbelief, embarrassment, guilt, and shame or may even fail to grasp how serious the problem is. Physical aggression is an emergency. All "usual" activities should be suspended until the episode passes. This is not the time to get someone dressed for bed, or insist on a shower.

- Keep the patient in full view. Any approach toward the patient (or vice versa) should be from the front, where both can watch each other. The patient should be given lots of space.

- The caregiver should be aware of his or her own body language. Remember, especially when verbal skills are compromised, that gestures mean a lot. Try to appear relaxed, and use a measured, low, soft voice to quiet the situation.
- While appearing to remain calm, be deliberate and in control. Use simple declarative sentences for directions, such as, "Give me the knife" or "Put the knife down."
- Reduce distractions in the area. Turn off the TV and radio and stop any extraneous stimuli.
- Even if the patient calms down, the risk remains. Violent gestures may be time-limited because of the energy expended, but after the patient rests, the violence can recur if the trigger remains. In cases of caregiver injury, there were often warnings, but the caregiver chose not to heed them, often out of disbelief that the loved one would ever hurt him or her.
- The caregiver should not stay alone in the house with a violent patient and should get help immediately. The family should call 911 and the patient should be handled by the emergency paramedics. The arrival of police or uniformed paramedics is sometimes calming for the patient, but medical care should still be sought as the episode may recur after they depart. If the problem is severe enough, inpatient treatment is warranted. If the violence was more threat and the danger level is felt to be minimal, outpatient treatment may still be appropriate, but this will usually entail pharmacotherapy as previously detailed.
- A Lifeline (panic button) to call for help may be helpful in homes where the risk of violence exists.
- The "safe escape contingency": Patients who are at risk of violent behavior remain a threat to their caregiver and family. In such homes, families should have an escape route, should be prepared to lock themselves away from a violent person, and should have a cellular phone handy.
- Violence is more likely to start at night, so caregivers may wish to move to another bedroom, one with a lock.
- Many things can be used as a weapon. As previously discussed, there should be no guns in the house, even in a locked cabinet. Fireplace pokers and knives should be stored out of sight. In panic, a book, alarm clock, letter opener, cane, or even a small table can cause injury.
- AD patients should not drive, but stopping them may be difficult. Under no circumstances should an angry or violent person drive, as the car can then become a weapon. If the patient takes the car to go out looking for a real or imaginary enemy, the police should be immediately notified.

References

1. Ouldred E, Bryant C. Dementia care, part 2: Understanding and managing behavioural challenges. Br J Nurs 2008;17(4):242–247.
2. Hall G. Testing the PLST Model with Community-Based Caregivers. Doctoral dissertation. Iowa City: University of Iowa, 1998.

3. Caron W, Boss P, Mortimer J. Family boundary ambiguity predicts Alzheimer's outcomes. Psychiatry 1999;62(4):347–356.

4. Cohen-Mansfield J, Jensen B. Assessment and treatment approaches for behavioral disturbances associated with dementia in the nursing home: self-reports of physicians' practices. Comment in: J Am Med Dir Assoc 2008;9(9):622–625.

5. Hall G, Buckwalter K. A conceptual model for planning and evaluating care of the client with Alzheimer's disease. Arch Psychiatric Nurs 1987;1(6):399–406.

6. Smith M, Hall G, Gerdner L, et al. Application of the Progressively Lowered Stress Threshold (PLST) model across the continuum of care. Nurs Clin North Am 2006;41(1):57–81.

7. Schulz R, O'Brien A, Ory M, et al. Dementia caregiver intervention research: In search of clinical significance. Gerontologist 2002;42:589–602.

Chapter 15

Planning ahead: legal issues and advance directives

The progressive nature of AD eventually renders patients unable to make responsible decisions about their finances and healthcare. Failing to prepare for the day when a loved one cannot make decisions can result in a host of unwelcome outcomes (even for the spouse):

- Bills may not be paid.
- Social Security problems will be difficult to resolve.
- Property and income taxes may not be paid appropriately or in a timely manner.
- Because of federal privacy laws, the family will be refused access to medical information, including when the person with dementia is hospitalized, has a sudden change in behavior, or has problems with medications.
- The person with dementia may be at increased risk for exploitation because he or she can still be convinced to sign contracts, charge items, or write checks.
- End-of-life decisions and care preferences will not be known and/or implemented.
- Banks, financial institutions, and insurance companies will refuse to work with the family.
- Another relative or total stranger may come in and obtain a power of attorney when the person with dementia does not understand what he or she is signing.
- Family members may become deeply divided by arguing what they feel is the best care for the person with dementia.

Starting the Discussion

A common fear of patients, which often worsens over time and which may adversely influence their decisions regarding their own healthcare and finances if not addressed early, is that their family will abandon them by placing them in a nursing home. One way to initiate a conversation about long-term care options is when a friend or relative requires care. Begin by discussing how the person with dementia feels about the friend's care and how (or if) he or she would do things differently. Extending the discussion to include all members of the household and what each would prefer should the need arise in each family member's own case lessens the sense of isolation and personal fear the patient feels. This may be more easily done early in the disease course when the decisions seem far in the future. Encourage the family to write down or otherwise document and preserve these preferences so they will be available for reference to guide future decisions.

Legal and Financial Affairs

Legal and financial issues should be addressed as early as possible. A husband or wife acting as caregiver may think that marriage entitles him or her to information about his or her spouse or gives him or her the right to make decisions on the loved one's behalf. Because federal laws on privacy now affect what healthcare, insurance, and banks and other financial institutions can disclose, spouses are not automatically entitled to information, nor are they automatically designated as substitute decision-makers. Most care for dementia is paid for out of pocket, so families must manage assets carefully. Gifts of money or property to adult children given with the intention of preserving assets for potential heirs are another common concern.

Families should be encouraged to consult with attorneys from the legal specialties of elder law, family law, or probate law. Standby durable powers of attorney for healthcare and finances should be developed for when the person is not able to make informed decisions. Additional decision-makers may need to be appointed for the patient in complex family financial situations. If there are business or agricultural concerns, additional legal expertise will be needed. The family members should be encouraged to seek legal counsel at their earliest convenience to ensure the patient's wishes are recorded and his or her estate preserved (1).

Healthcare Proxy and Advance Directives

Patients with dementia as well as their caregivers both need advance directives, as even caregivers can become ill and die first. Laws for healthcare proxies vary from state to state. Many states have this information online, or it may be obtained from the local chapter of the Alzheimer's Association (http://www.alz.org/apps/findus.asp) (2).

A temporary healthcare proxy can be appointed, usually by completing a relatively simple form designating who can be provided with ongoing medical information if the patient becomes impaired, in which case the proxy is empowered to make decisions on the patient's behalf. However, once the patient becomes severely and permanently impaired as a result of progressive and irreversible dementia, then durable medical power of attorney (DPOA) is required. DPOA means that the power of attorney remains in effect despite the person's cognitive impairments. In some states a physician must provide a written statement attesting to the patient's impairment before a DPOA can be enacted. (Some states also have durable mental health power of attorney. These DPOAs allow a designee to make decisions about mental health treatment, including the decision for involuntary hospitalization, and to communicate with mental health providers.) A copy of the DPOA should be kept in all medical and hospital records. In most states there is no scheduled oversight of people designated as DPOAs, and providers suspecting exploitation are required to report such concerns to the state's adult protective services.

Living wills are a form of advance directive that offer the patient the opportunity to establish and communicate the values by which he or she would like major medical decisions made in the event of incapacity and in specific scenarios, such as whether resuscitation should be attempted following a cardiorespiratory arrest; a feeding tube placed if the patient is unable to eat; or intubation performed for respiratory failure. Living wills can be established with fairly simple forms and should be kept in a health file at home as well in all relevant medical records (3,4).

Guardianship and Conservatorship

If a patient has failed to designate a DPOA, and/or legal or psychiatric issues arise, the family may need to pursue either of two options that are granted by the court: guardianship gives the designee parent-like responsibilities over the patient; conservatorship provides the designee responsibilities for the patient's estate.

Both options can be either voluntary, where the patient signs in agreement with the petition, or involuntary, where the patient is judged by the court to be incapacitated. Specific laws governing guardianship and conservatorship vary from state to state, but in all states guardians and conservators are appointed and monitored by the court. Guardians must account at least annually about how they are meeting the physical, emotional, and social needs of the patient. Conservators must account for all financial transactions (3,4).

Applying for involuntary conservatorship and/or guardianship can be long, involved, and costly as there are multiple attorneys involved, physician evaluations, and at least one hearing. It is also stressful because the petitioner is placed in an adversarial relationship with the patient until the court announces its findings. In many states guardians must petition the court in order to make changes, especially for relocating the patient. Some states have laws for emergency guardianship where a temporary appointment can be made. This is often done when the patient is determined to be at high risk for injury or has developed psychosis.

Determining Capacity

Primary care physicians are often called upon, whether explicitly or implicitly (meaning they find themselves held accountable in medicolegal situations when the patient has acted inappropriately and the question arises as to whether the doctor informed the patient and family of the patient's incapacity), to determine the patient's capacity to make decisions, drive, manage money, and safely live alone. This is often difficult for several reasons:

- The patient's mental status fluctuates throughout the day and week
- The provider has relatively little time to observe the patient and provide a thoughtful opinion
- The provider must rely on accompanying family members, who are often uneducated in dementia and perhaps resistant to mentioning the extent of the problem in front of the patient
- There are few objective generally available assessments to determine capacity
- The provider may not have access to behavioral neurology, geriatric psychiatry, and/or neuropsychological testing for referrals
- Medicare and third-party payers may resist paying for referrals to determine capacity

Studies of patient awareness in dementia have conflicting findings. One study of 80 people with moderate to advanced dementia reported that all 80 subjects demonstrated awareness of their conditions at least some of the time, yet two thirds also had periods when they were not aware (5). Awareness, however, does not translate into decision-making capacity. The legal standard of capacity requires "demonstrating understanding, appreciation, reasoning and stating a choice" (6). Even patients with MCI perform significantly below controls on the three clinically relevant standards of appreciation, reasoning, and understanding (7). Unfortunately, for most legal purposes there is no "partial capacity."

There are several avenues a provider may use to determine a patient's mental capacity:

- Patient and family reports of functional abilities of instrumental activities, paying particular attention to reports of problems with finances (paying bills, being scammed or exploited, changes in spending habits), shopping, experiencing psychosis (especially paranoia), driving (mishaps, fender-benders, traffic citations, needing a co-pilot, getting lost, refusing to give up driving despite obvious hazards), and issues of living alone (not eating, house filled with trash, barricading self in the house, neighbors complaining, 911 calls, police involvement)
- Assessment of reading comprehension by providing an article or anecdote for the patient to read. Once the patient has read the article and handed it back, ask what the written piece was about. If the patient replies, "I wasn't paying attention" or "It wasn't very interesting," suspect he or she is trying to compensate for a lack of reading comprehension.

- Objective assessment of mental status: this can be as simple as performing a MMSE, although if the patient exhibits deficits in attention and executive function indicative of frontal lobe involvement, he or she may score well (8).
- If there are conflicting or ambiguous data from the first three sources, a referral for neuropsychological testing should be made. The request must be specific: "Does this patient have capacity to make decisions about his or her care (drive? live alone?)." This cues the psychologist to test for the necessary information and assists with the judgment. Neuropsychological testing is especially important (and recommended) in medicolegal settings, and during earlier disease stages when incapacity may not be obvious.

Community Resources

Relevant community resources available to patients and families include the Alzheimer's Association and the area agency on aging. The Alzheimer's Association has chapters all over the United States and offers a variety of services for both patients and families (2). Educational programs include the nature and course of AD, legal and financial planning, dealing with specific problems, and community resources that are available and how to access them. They usually hold support groups for affected families and have a wide array of written and video-based learning materials, often available in other languages.

Area agencies on aging are located throughout the United States and are easily found by searching online for: "Area Agency on Aging, County, and State" (e.g., "Area Agency on Aging, Johnson County, Iowa"). These agencies provide access to most of the community resources in a given area and can advise families on available public funding and how and where to apply.

References

1. Fisher Center for Alzheimer's Research Foundation. Legal and Financial Planning. 2008; accessed April 13, 2009. Available at: http://www.alzinfo.org/alzheimers-legal-financial.asp

2. Alzheimer's Association Chapter Finder. Retrieved April 10, 2009, from http://www.alz.org/apps/findus.asp

3. Fisher Center for Alzheimer's Research Foundation. Alzheimer's Resources: Power of Attorney. 2008; accessed April 13, 2009. Available at: http://www.alzinfo.org/alzheimers-power-attorney.asp#1

4. National Institute on Aging. Legal & Financial Planning for People with Alzheimer's Disease. National Institute of Health, 2007; accessed April 13, 2009. Available at: http://www.nia.nih.gov/Alzheimers/Publications/legaltips.htm

5. Clare L, Rowlands J, Bruce E, et al. "I don't do like I used to do": a grounded theory approach to conceptualizing awareness in people with moderate to severe dementia living in long-term care. Social Science & Medicine 2008;66(11):2366–2377. Accessed April 14, 2009. Available at: http://ovidsp.ovid.com/ovidweb.cgi?T=JS&NEWS=N&PAGE=fulltext&AN=18325650&D=medl

6. Rodin MB, Mohile SG. Assessing decisional capacity in the elderly. Semin Oncol 2008;35(6):625–632.

7. Okonkwo OC, Griffith HR, Copeland JN, et al. Medical decision-making capacity in mild cognitive impairment: a 3-year longitudinal study. Neurology 2008;71(19):1474–1480.

8. Pezzotti P, Scalmana S, Mastromattei A, et al. The accuracy of the MMSE in detecting cognitive impairment when administered by general practitioners: a prospective observational study. BMC Family Practice 2008;9:29.

Chapter 16

The long-term care continuum

Because AD is a lifelong condition, care is necessarily "long term," but there is a continuum that ranges from simple companionship in the earliest stages to nursing home care (or its in-home equivalent) in late stages. In the mild and moderate disease stages families can consider adult day programming ("adult day healthcare"). These are certified programs that offer structured group activities and often lunch. Even when patients seem satisfied with caregiver companionship, it is often beneficial for the caregiver to have some "away time." Adult day healthcare is an ideal first step in seeking services. After an "initiation period" in which the caregiver accompanies the patient for two days, most (but not all) patients settle in to programs and look forward to going. Many programs offer transportation and some more personalized care. Most states require a physician's order and tuberculin test (or chest x-ray) for admission to adult day programming. Research suggests that patients who participate in adult day programming are more engaged, have fewer behavioral problems, and adapt more readily to institutionalization (when necessary) later.

Services for people with dementia differ from those offered to people who are physically frail. Frail people need assistance with physical care but can determine and express their preferences for activities. For patients with dementia, activities are the focus of programming, with physical care being incidental. Dementia-specific programming is concerned with managing fatigue; providing consistency, socialization, and staff contact; managing stimuli; and helping patients to participate in and enjoy a variety of planned activities throughout the day. Families should ask about the number of hours of dementia-specific training each employee receives, observe staff interacting with patients, and ask about family participation in the program. Whenever given a choice of a dementia-specific program versus an "integrated program that also has some people with dementia," they should be encouraged to select the former.

Home-Based Care

Home care is generally provided by agencies that offer "respite" or "companion services" and is paid for out of pocket. Some services, such as visiting nurses, are less appropriate for people with dementia due to strict Medicare guidelines for "short-term, intermittent, skilled care to people who are home-bound." Some patients with long-term care insurance have benefits that include in-home care. Caregivers should be encouraged to review their policies with a care manager (trained social worker or nurse) to determine whether their policy will pay for in-home services.

Triggers for placement in an institution include safety concerns, wandering, inability to take medications properly, inability to manage food, lack of personal care, becoming frightened, incontinence, psychosis, or repeated falls. Patients who live alone will suffer these problems earlier than those living with others but may do quite well after placement. For those receiving care at home, the trigger is usually that care needs exceed what can be provided, incontinence, severe sleep disturbance, and/or significant behavioral problems. Another reason for placement is the illness or death of the caregiver. There are a wide variety of residential living options (Table 16.1).

Adult Foster Homes

Adult foster care homes typically provide care for up to four people, and the caregiver lives in the home. Assisted living homes are individual homes where care is provided for up to about 10 people. In both cases, there may be around-the-clock personnel who are not trained clinicians but can provide basic personal care and supervision. There are no formal programs of care, there may or may not be activities, and there is no medical supervision.

Table 16.1 Residential Care Options

Group Homes	Assisted Living	Nursing Homes
No formal program of care	Can be anything	Regulated by state & fed rules
No staff training or requirements	May have no staff requirements or training (depends on state)	Requirements for number of personnel, training, ongoing education
Few have specific memory care focus	May not have memory care program	May not have memory care program
Very limited state oversight May change meds as caregiver sees fit	Medical oversight may be very limited	Careful medication and medical oversight
No professionals onsite	May not be professionals onsite (anyone is called "the nurse")	Have RNs and MD oversight
May not have activities	May not have activities or may have general activities for frail people (e.g., bingo)	Have mandated activities yet based on medical model

Assisted Living Facilities

Assisted living facilities (ALFs) care for larger numbers of people but most of the other attributes are the same. In most ALFs the care contract is simply a rental agreement. As a general rule, patients rent an apartment. Most ALFs offer one or more meals per day (some charge extra for this) and intermittent light housekeeping. Supervision, medication administration, and personal care are available but contracted separately. Personnel may or may not have any specific training in dementia care. Government oversight is relatively limited. "Directed care" ("ALF memory care") is specialized memory care that can be provided in any of these settings; it requires additional certification and training (1).

Many ALFs have specialized memory care units specifically for people with dementia. These units are often secured to prevent wandering and will be more likely to offer activities designed for people with cognitive impairment. Families will often initially reject memory care, thinking the patient will be fine in the standard ALF apartments, but often patients decompensate on admission due to relocation trauma and must be quickly moved to memory care. It is best to advise families to consider memory care first.

Skilled Nursing Facilities

Skilled nursing facilities provide a higher level of care for people who are truly dependent in basic activities of daily living such as bathing, dressing, eating, and toileting and/or require daily medical nursing care. Personnel have specified training and certification, and these facilities are regulated by state and federal officials. There are nurses and physicians on site. There may or may not be formal memory programs; activity programs are mandated but may be based on medical models not well suited to people with dementia.

Choosing the right setting requires understanding the specifics of each option. On-site visits are necessary to compare and contrast. We recommend that families ask questions of staff as well as residents and family members. Do staff articulate and practice the "high-touch, low-tech" approach to providing memory care? Do they understand what makes their residents comfortable or stressed? Are the residents clean? Often the best facilities will have lower staff turnover and higher staff satisfaction and morale, which we view as more important than cosmetic amenities (2).

It is important for families to understand that as a general rule Medicare does not pay for any residential or adult day services for people with dementia because services are considered "custodial," not skilled. If the family members believe the patient's resources will be depleted, they must go to their Department of Human Services and apply for Title 19 (Medicaid) coverage. The earlier the family applies, the more resources a spouse will be able to keep. Services covered by Medicaid vary from state to state. The Alzheimer's Association can advise families of what is covered in the person's state.

References

1. Smith M, Buckwalter K, Kang H, et al. Dementia care in assisted living: Needs and challenges. Issues inMental Health Nursing 2008;29:8:817–838.

2. Casarett D, Takesaka J, Karlawish J, et al. How should clinicians discuss hospice for patients with dementia? Anticipating caregivers' preconceptions and meeting their information needs. Alzheimer Dis Assoc Disord 2002;16(2):116–122.

Chapter 17

End-of-life care for dementia

End-of-life care for patients with advanced dementia is an important aspect of medical care as patients with advanced dementia, often residing in nursing facilities, frequently live from 1 to 3 years. AD and related dementias are the sixth leading cause of death in the United States, with 67% of deaths occurring in long-term care facilities (1,2). During this final phase of illness, patients with advanced dementia have severe cognitive impairment (MMSE < 10), are unable to ambulate without maximum assistance, cannot communicate in a meaningful fashion, and require assistance for all activities of daily living. Preceding death, most patients will develop recurrent infections and/or fever and be prone to weight loss and pressure ulcers. Less than 10% of patients with advanced dementia receive hospice care, and only recently have palliative care measures been considered in this much-compromised population (3). This may reflect that many physicians, long-term care providers, and families do not think of dementia as a terminal illness so that comfort measures are not implemented until death is imminent. Furthermore, it is very challenging for physicians to prognosticate the final 6 months of life as required when using the hospice Medicare benefit (4). Consequently, many patients with advanced dementia are subject to uncomfortable interventions ranging from lab draws to artificial feedings, mechanical restraints, and/or hospitalization (5). Physicians can play a key role in ensuring maximum comfort for the patient and facilitating important discussions with family caregivers about medical treatment and care.

Symptom Management

There are many recognized discomforts related to advanced dementia, including pain, skin breakdown, falls, contractures, incontinence, dysphagia, and weight loss (5,6). When other coexisting chronic diseases are taken into consideration as well, it becomes both obvious and imperative to focus on comfort treatments and modalities because patients with advanced dementia lack the verbal and cognitive skills to report discomfort. Consequently, many of the behavioral disturbances reported or observed in this population are due to unmet physiological or basic needs. A need-driven, dementia-compromised behavior model (7) provides a framework for behaviors to be viewed as a symptom of unmet needs in the patient's attempt to communicate either physical or psychic distress.

Need-driven behaviors can be challenging to interpret in the patient with advanced dementia and may be ignored or even perceived as normal for that individual. For example, many caregivers report that it is difficult to distinguish behaviors related to physical pain versus hunger or the psychic pain related to frustration in daily living. When basic needs are left unaddressed and/or unattended, behaviors may accelerate and are likely to be viewed as the problem, rather than the symptom of the problem. The consequences of seeing the behavior as a problem rather than the symptom are likely to result in ineffective treatment and added discomfort.

Pain

Pain is a common source of an unmet need in patients with advanced dementia (8,9). Despite changes in the brain from these neurodegenerative diseases, patients with advanced dementia can still experience pain sensations similar to that of cognitively intact patients (10). Common pain behaviors can result in resistance to care, agitation, restlessness, and physical aggression. Other pain-related behaviors may include nonverbal features such as frowning, facial grimacing, and tense and guarded body language. Verbalization of pain may present with moaning, crying, and other distressing vocalizations such as yelling. Daily living patterns may also be affected in patients who stop eating or participating in favorite activities (9). Immobility and osteoarthritic pain are the most common sources of pain in the population; however, it is not uncommon for these individuals to have unrecognized fractures. It is well documented that pain is poorly assessed in long-term care settings and analgesia is often ordered as needed rather than on a scheduled basis. In acute care settings, it has been suggested that patients with advanced dementia receive significantly less attention to pain and therefore significantly less pain medication (11). The results of pain-related behaviors and unscheduled medications indicate that patients with advanced dementia are undertreated for pain; interventions are needed to improve pain detection and management (12).

Assessing pain as the fifth vital sign recognizes that all patients with pain deserve to have prompt recognition and treatment and that pain needs to be routinely assessed, monitored, and documented in all healthcare settings. While some patients with advanced dementia may be able to report a simple "yes/no" or vocalize pain, most will be unable to do so. A number of behavioral assessment tools have been developed to identify pain in patients with advanced dementia (13–18). While there is no consensus regarding which of these tools is best to assess for pain, a convenient one for clinicians is the Pain Assessment in Advanced Dementia (PAINAD) Scale (13) (Table 17.1).

Observed pain behaviors are not always accurate reflections of pain intensity. When a behavioral tool is used, the score should not be interpreted as a pain intensity rating as compared with standard pain scales. Rather, the

Table 17.1 Pain Assessment in Dementia Scale				
	0	**1**	**2**	**Score**
Breathing	Normal	Occasional labored Brief hyperventilation	Noisy labored Extended hyperventilation; Cheyne-Stokes respiration	
Negative vocalization	None	Occasional moan Low-level disapproving verbalization	Repeated calling, yelling, or crying Loud moaning	
Facial expression	Smiling Inexpressive	Sad, frightened	Grimacing	
Body language	Relaxed	Tense; pacing; fidgeting	Rigid; clenched fists; striking out	
Consolability	No need to console	Distracted or reassured by touch/voice	Unable to distract, console, or reassure	

Each item is scored from 0 to 2 for a total score of 0 to 10. Scores over 4 are interpreted to mean the patient is in pain and requires a treatment plan. Reprinted from Warden V, Hurley AC, Volicer L. Development and psychometric evaluation of the Pain Assessment in Advanced Dementia (PAINAD) scale. Journal of the American Medical Directors Association 2003;4(1):9–15. Copyright 2003, with permission from Elsevier.

behavioral assessment tools are most helpful to identify the presence of pain and to evaluate the effectiveness of treatment (8,9,12).

Recent practice recommendations provide consistent and practical strategies to assess and manage pain in this population (8,19). Despite cognitive impairment, attempts should be made to ascertain the presence of pain from the patient. Patients are more likely to respond "yes/no" when the clinician holds his or her hand over a potentially painful site or asks the patient to point to what hurts. When that technique is not possible, the next step is to employ behavioral assessment. Each physician and/or facility should adopt a behavioral assessment tool that is used consistently to quantify behaviors. In the absence of stated pain, the behavioral assessment is a valid approach, using a score to establish the presence of discomfort as well as determining if pain interventions are effective when implemented. Surrogate reports of pain from family caregivers or staff may also be helpful but should not be used alone as they may be inconsistent among caregivers.

When basic physiological needs such as hunger, thirst, toileting and positioning have been met and the behavioral assessment indicates discomfort, it should be assumed that pain is present. The next step in effective pain management is searching for potential causes of pain. Chronic pain conditions should be considered and assessed along with any recent changes, such as falls, infections, and skin tears.

Attempts to manage pain with analgesics and nonpharmacological measures should then be employed. When pain is considered mild to moderate, acetaminophen 500 to 1,000 mg every 6 hours may be appropriate, not exceeding 3 grams per 24 hours. If pain behaviors continue per the identified behavioral assessment tool, titration to stronger analgesics is warranted. Low-dose opioids have been effective in decreasing agitation as an indicator of pain. However, initial opioid doses should be reduced by 25% to 50% in older patients (20). It is essential to provide an adequate analgesia trial before adding psychotropic medications. Typically, the response to an analgesic intervention can be seen fairly quickly and any sedative properties due to analgesics will not obscure pain. When opioids are used, it is essential to add a stool softener. Effective use of pain medication will require that medications are scheduled and adjusted as needed, and ongoing assessment is crucial. If pain medications alone do not improve behaviors, adding or changing doses of antipsychotics, antidepressants, or sedatives may be needed (5,8,9,19).

Finally, the use of nonpharmacological measures can bring additional comfort and support for the patient with advanced dementia. Gentle touch, light massage, a warm compress, favorite music, and repositioning are all effective methods that should be used by caregivers in addition to analgesia (9).

Skin Disorders and Breakdown

Skin disorders and breakdown, including pressure ulcers, are common in patients with advanced dementia due to immobility, incontinence, and poor hydration and nutrition (21). Moreover, skin breakdown is often associated with pain. It is essential that all precautions are taken when stage 1 redness appears. Daily skin assessment, especially over vulnerable areas such as the hips and coccyx, is imperative. Ensuring that the patient is repositioned every 2 hours and has frequent continent care, along with accurate documentation, will assist in preventing pressure ulcers. Topical moisture is good preventive care when applied gently and without massage over bony areas. Special attention should be given when moving a patient in bed or during transfers from bed to wheelchair, as skin friction may lead to shearing and/or skin tears. A wound care specialist can also be helpful in providing other prevention techniques and treatment plans when stage 2 to 4 pressure ulcers are present.

Nutrition

Nutritional problems are common in advanced dementia and can result in weight loss, dehydration, and aspiration. However, patients with advanced dementia can live for long periods of time despite poor oral intake: it has been theorized that there is a reduced metabolic rate, resulting in lower caloric intake, along with altered homeostasis (22). Eating problems often begin as the patient loses the ability to feed himself or herself; this is usually the last activity of daily living lost prior to death. Many patients will forget to chew or chew continuously, with a greater tendency to pocket food or spit foods that are not pleasurable. Swallowing problems may be due to delayed initiation or multiple swallows, making aspiration much more likely to occur. Other common reasons for decreased food intake include depression and lack of interest in food; overstimulating environments, leading to an inability to focus on the meal;

fatigue; ill-fitting dentures; and acute illness (23). Recent studies of dining strategies for patients with advanced dementia provide overwhelming evidence that providing small frequent meals and focusing on taste and texture are extremely important factors in getting patients to accept and swallow food (23,24).

A customized dining program using hand feeding should be the treatment of choice for patients with eating problems. The goal is to maintain continued oral feeding so that it provides a comfortable and pleasurable eating experience. However, hand feeding is labor-intensive, requiring approximately 45 to 90 minutes per day, and poor staffing can be a barrier to effective dining programs (24). A customized program requires that favorite foods be readily available 24 hours per day, with soft and sweet snacks offered between meals and at bedtime. It is becoming more common for staff to eat with patients, as they can provide an example of how to eat and can carefully observe the patient during dining. All of these efforts can be effective in minimizing weight loss (25).

There are multiple benefits to hand feeding. Patients can continue to enjoy the pleasure of food, and it is often one of the most important daily activities experienced in a long-term care setting. Mealtimes allow for interaction between the patient and the staff and/or family caregivers. Feeding the patient can provide a meaningful role for family members, as they can also bring in favorite foods for the person to enjoy. It is not uncommon for patients to eat favorite foods up to the final weeks of life when customized dining practices are put into place (25,26).

Feeding tubes are considered another approach to managing eating problems. It has been estimated that almost 30% of advanced dementia patients in the United States have feeding tubes, particularly those who are younger, those who are African American, those who lack advance directives, and those who reside in a Medicaid-reimbursed facility (25–27). While feeding tubes have been thought to prolong life, improve nutrition, prevent aspiration and pressure sores, and promote comfort, there is mounting evidence that none of these benefits are supported. Rather, studies now suggest that survival is not improved; nutritional status is not enhanced; pressure sores are not less prevalent; aspiration may be more common; and physical restraints are more likely to be used to prevent removal of the feeding tube, thus leading to greater discomfort (5,6,24,26,27). Moreover, families report lower satisfaction with end-of-life care when patients with advanced dementia have feeding tubes (28). Hence, the physician plays a key role in promoting comfort with eating problems and in the prevention of feeding tubes by thoughtful discussion with family and professional caregivers about the benefits of careful hand feeding and the evidence of morbidity caused by tube feeding.

Immobility and Falls

Immobility and falls are common in advanced dementia. Patients have poor insight and judgment, along with neurological motor changes. However, the need to move is often primal in these individuals, making them at great risk for falls. Despite growing litigation over falls, physical restraints should be used very judiciously as other behaviors are likely to occur when the person's movement is limited: increased physical agitation and yelling may result, leading to requests from caregivers for antipsychotics. Maximizing mobility is very effective in both preventing falls and promoting comfort in this population. Caregivers may need instruction to anticipate the patient's need for movement and assist the patient throughout the day with sit-to-stand motions and simple short steps. This will often alleviate the need for physical restraints, as the patient's need for movement is satisfied throughout the day. A physical therapist can be extremely helpful in teaching caregivers to implement a preventive program. Patients must have good footwear with nonskid soles, and foot care/nail care is necessary for comfort in wearing shoes.

Contractures

Contractures and frozen joints can result from disuse and immobility. Range of motion should be performed as part of a daily activity pattern, along with adequate pain management measures. Splinting of joints and contractures may also be necessary to ensure maximal comfort. As the patient spends more of the day sitting in a chair or lying in bed, special attention should be given to positioning. Chair dimensions should fit the patient without the need for pillows or constant adjustment. The patient should comfortably be able to self-propel; thus, shorter patients should not have their legs dangling without touching the floor. The chair seat height is determined by the length of the patient's lower leg, the seat depth by the thigh length, the seat width by hip width, and the back height by fit to the person's head and back. Some patients require a customized chair. Likewise, the bed height should allow the patient to sit on the edge of the bed with his or her feet flat of the floor. Low beds are often available in many assisted living or skilled nursing facilities. Occasionally a mattress will be placed directly on the floor if the patient is impulsive and has a history of falls. Bed alarms can be used but may have limitations in warning caregivers of the patient's movement from bed. The alarm itself may also be frightening to an already confused person.

Incontinence

Urinary and fecal incontinence in advanced dementia requires special care. Indwelling catheters should be avoided as they cause discomfort for the patient and pose a greater risk for infection. Some patients can successfully void on the toilet when toileting programs are employed. However, caregivers must be motivated to take the patient to the toilet every 2 to 3 hours. Disposable briefs are commonly used and should be changed immediately after soiling to prevent skin irritation and breakdown.

Many patients with advanced dementia can maintain fecal continence when the caregiver places the patient comfortably on the commode, keeping with the patient's normal pattern. This not only provides dignity to the patient but can decrease much of the agitation seen in patients needing to defecate. These individuals are at risk for constipation due to decreased fluid and food intake coupled with immobility. Fecal impaction is not uncommon and may present as diarrhea when it is overflow fecal incontinence. Other symptoms may include abdominal tenderness, distention, and a mass in the lower left quadrant of the abdomen. Prevention of constipation is best managed using natural agents such as prunes or prune juice and by adding fiber to the diet. Stool softeners can be helpful along with mild stimulating agents. Low-volume phosphate enemas should be the treatment of choice for fecal impaction, followed by digital manipulation should several enemas be unsuccessful.

Dyspnea

Dyspnea, typically secondary to pneumonia, is another common symptom in end-of-life dementia care. While treatment of pneumonia and infections in advanced dementia are discussed later in the chapter, it has been suggested that dyspnea and pain are often associated with pneumonia and must be targeted to achieve maximal comfort care (29). While treatment of infections with antimicrobials may play a role in the treatment of dyspnea, more conservative treatment, including the use of oxygen, analgesics, and antipyretics, must consistently be employed (24,29,30).

Medical Care

As the focus of care is directed at comfort in advanced dementia, physicians must rethink many of the standard interventions that have been used up to this time. Management of medical issues must be based on well-defined treatment goals in conjunction with the family/medical decision-maker, while avoiding treatment decisions that provide little benefit and impose greater discomfort on the patient. Aggressive medical interventions will cause greater discomfort in those with advanced dementia, as their ability to understand and cooperate with the therapeutic intervention is severely compromised. Thus, the burden of therapeutic interventions is greater in this population than in cognitively intact patients (5). Even routine procedures such as blood pressure measurement and blood sugar testing may cause behavioral symptoms and distress. Preventive measures such as cancer screening/detection and those used to tightly control a chronic disease such as diabetes provide little value.

Therapeutic use of medications used to treat dementia and other chronic illnesses deserves special consideration as the focus moves away from disease modification to management of symptoms and comfort care (31). Polypharmacy is present in many of these patients, who cannot verbalize symptoms, and this can contribute to unwanted side effects, including dizziness, sedation, constipation, and further cognitive decline (32). While few studies have addressed appropriate prescribing in advanced dementia, some studies have established that patients often receive inappropriate medications, and one recent study demonstrated that one in four advanced dementia patients received antipsychotic medications at the end of life (6,31). Therefore, an appropriate strategy for physicians should be to simplify the medication regimen whenever possible. All medications should be carefully reviewed for appropriateness, eliminating agents that have limited benefit. For example, discontinuing lipid-lowering medications and osteoporosis medications, minimizing cardiac medications, and so forth may be beneficial for the patient dying from advanced dementia. Minimizing the number of medications will also assist in avoiding drug reactions and interactions. Finally, while donepezil and memantine are now FDA approved for advanced AD, when the patient is bedbound and no longer able to feed himself or herself, it is reasonable to consider discontinuing these therapies. A thoughtful discussion should occur with the family and/or medical power of attorney regarding appropriate medication use at the end of life, with decisions reflecting the stated goals of care (5,31,32).

Physicians play a key role in the avoidance of emergency department use and hospitalization in advanced dementia, particularly when transfer is due to infection or breathing difficulties. This is an important aspect to good medical care, as both of these settings are overstimulating and stressful for these patients and can impose a significant degree of risk with limited benefits. It has been demonstrated that over one third of unscheduled transfers from nursing facilities to the emergency department and hospital were inappropriate for residents with advanced dementia (33). In fact, good medical care can be rendered in most long-term care facilities while minimizing burden to the patient. Data now support that optimal treatment of patients with pneumonia in nursing facilities has better long-term outcomes than hospital treatment (5,24). Thus, hospitalization should be considered only when it is consistent with the overall goals of care for the patient.

Healthcare Decisions in Advanced Dementia

Implicit to good medical care is continued discussion with the family and particularly the appointed medical power of attorney about medical care. Families often lack information that is necessary in end-of-life decision making. Advance directives are often incomplete or absent and rarely reflect previously stated patient preferences. Most families are unaware about the progression of dementia and do not know what to expect at the end of life. Most are unaware that pneumonia is the most common cause of death and that administration of antimicrobials may not be consistent with the goals of care.

Ideally, discussions about healthcare decisions for dementia should occur in earlier stages of the disease, when the patient has the capacity to participate and provide guidance to family members (34). However, most patients and families do not have the discussion, and families are left to make important end-of-life decisions. Healthcare decisions unique to advanced dementia include the use of antibiotics to treat infections, use of feeding tubes and/or intravenous hydration, and hospitalization. Discussions should be ongoing; they may evoke much emotion, as family members often differ in opinions and treatment goals.

In the absence of a medical power of attorney, a surrogate decision-maker may make decisions. While each state has differing laws, surrogate decision-makers can include a spouse, adult child, sibling, domestic partner, or friend. The surrogate is responsible for making decisions that are consistent with what he or she believes the patient would want. It is often helpful during treatment discussions to ask the family or appointed decision maker, "If the patient could stand at the foot of the bed and see the situation as it is now, what would the patient tell you to do? Would he/she say to keep him/her comfortable by not prolonging her life in any way? Or would he/she say, please use every possible means to keep me alive?"

While the majority of older adults would not want CPR if they had severe dementia (35), it is not uncommon for families to select more life-sustaining measures. One study showed that spouses of patients with advanced dementia were more likely to forgo CPR, respirator use, and tube feeding, but only 10% of them would decline antibiotics. Families are much more comfortable consenting to treatment than they are with the decision to forgo treatment (36). These data support that it is imperative for physicians to have ongoing discussions as new problems arise. Conversations must provide education about treatment choices in the face of progressive disease while extending emotional support to families in their decision-making efforts.

Family Support

Both the challenges and consequences of caring for a patient with dementia are well documented. Caregivers consistently report high levels of stress, depression, and burden. Furthermore, caregivers are at greater risk for premature death as a result of the daily demands (1,37). Grief is often the core of the caregiving experience and is frequently overlooked or mislabeled as depression or stress by health professionals. Anticipatory grief may be useful for physicians to conceptualize the experience of dementia caregivers as they mourn the loss of what was, what is, and what will be over a prolonged period of time. Consequently, there are a wide range of emotions, thoughts, physical sensations, and behaviors that are encountered by caregivers as an extension of this experience. Caregiver grief in dementia can result from the personal sacrifices made by caregivers to meet the patient's growing daily care needs. There is often personal sadness about the effects of the disease on the patient and the longing for the relationship as it was prior to the disease. Many caregivers experience a depression-like sense of uncertainty, not knowing what the future holds for them or the patient. And it is common for caregivers to become isolated from family and friends or to withdraw altogether (37,38).

Spousal caregivers have different patterns of grief and loss as compared to adult children and thus may report differing thoughts and emotions when speaking of the effects of caregiving to the physician. Spouses experience gradual increases in their grief over the course of the disease. By the advanced stage of dementia, spouses tend to have feelings of sadness along with uncertainty about their own future, as they no longer feel like a couple but rather a single person. Thoughts of loneliness and general emptiness are also expressed. When the patient is moved to a facility, the caregiver often experiences extreme grief, stress, and guilt. Sadly, these caregivers are at greatest risk for depression following the death of the patient compared to caregivers who render care in the home (37).

In contrast to spousal caregivers, adult children often feel the highest level of grief during the moderate stage of dementia. It is during this time when they may be actively caring for a parent in addition to balancing other demands such as family and work. As a result, adult children may have feelings of anger, guilt, and resentment. By the stage of advanced dementia, adult children have greater feelings of sadness and regret related to the loss of relationship they feel with the parent. Typically, their level of grief dissipates as the parent is placed in a facility.

As the physician cares for the patient, it is important to check in with the family caregiver regarding his or her emotional health. While antidepressants may help the caregiver with depression and/or anxiety, overlooking the role of grief may interfere with the caregiver's coping and healing. It is essential to validate caregiving efforts and appreciate efforts to maintain connection to the patient. Support groups provided by the Alzheimer's Association (www.alz.org) and even grief groups often provided by hospice programs can be extremely helpful in assisting caregivers to cope with grief and loss. For those weary of groups, encouraging them to share feelings with a friend or confidant can be just as beneficial. Some caregivers may benefit by keeping a journal of their thoughts, feelings, and lessons learned. Others have benefited from more creative means, such as writing poetry or putting together a scrapbook of favorite pictures and recording memories. These memory books can be therapeutic for family and friends to remember the patient with dementia the way he or she was prior to developing the disease. The book can also help professional caregivers to better understand the person they are caring for. Finally, the physician should encourage the caregiver to maintain friendships, hobbies, and other activities outside of the caregiving duties, not only to promote respite time but also to prepare for a life following caregiving (39).

For those providing care to the patient in the home, the physician should provide assistance by connecting caregivers to respite care via in-home care agencies or through short-term respite options. A social worker, a private geriatric care manager, or a call to the local Alzheimer's Association can help connect caregivers to these valuable resources. When placement is required in a residential setting, families can use these same resources to locate a facility that best suits the patient's needs.

Hospice Care

AD as a terminal illness dictates that hospice care is warranted at the end of life, yet only about 10% of patients with dementia ever receive hospice care (1,5,6). Table 17.2 outlines the Medicare requirements for admission to hospice with a primary diagnosis of dementia (40).

Table 17.2 Hospice Eligibility for Dementia

Must show the following characteristics:
- Stage 7 or beyond according to the Functional Assessment Staging (FAST) Scale
- Unable to ambulate without assistance
- Unable to dress without assistance
- Unable to bathe without assistance
- Urinary and fecal incontinence, intermittent or constant
- No meaningful verbal communication; stereotypical phrases only or ability to speak is limited to six or fewer intelligible words

In addition, the patients must have had one of the following within the past 12 months:
- Aspiration pneumonia
- Pyelonephritis or other upper urinary tract infection
- Septicemia
- Decubitus ulcers, multiple, stage 3 or 4
- Fever, recurrent after antibiotics
- Inability to maintain sufficient fluid and calorie intake, with 10% weight loss during the previous 6 months, or serum albumin is <2 g/dL

While these requirements are not good predictors of death in 6 months or less, applying these guidelines allows physicians to begin discussion with the family about the use of hospice care. Hospice can provide important services for both the patient and the family and it is best applied before death is imminent.

It has been documented that advanced dementia patients receiving hospice care are twice as likely to receive treatment of pain and other symptoms than non-hospice patients (41). The hospice team provides additional comprehensive assessment to ensure overall patient comfort. The team comprises a nurse, certified nursing assistant, social worker, chaplain, and volunteer. In addition to comfort measures provided by the nurse and certified nursing assistant, the chaplain can facilitate familiar and favorite spiritual practices and the social worker can provide opportunities for sensory stimulation. The social worker and chaplain can provide needed support, counseling, and spiritual care for the caregiver along with bereavement counseling following the death of the patient. Caregivers often report that the hospice benefit is more helpful to them than to the patient (42).

In summary, caring for the patient at the end of life is challenging and requires the physician to maximize comfort through good symptom management, prudent attention to medical care issues, decreasing burden of treatment to the patient, continued discussions about healthcare decisions, supporting the caregiver with the grief experience, and prompt referral to hospice care for support before and after death.

References

1. Alzheimer's Association. 2009 Alzheimer's disease facts and figures. Alzheimers Dementia 2009;5(3):234–270.

2. Mitchell SL, Teno JM, Miller SC, et al. A national study of the location of death for older persons with dementia. J Am Geriatr Soc 2005;53:299–305.

3. Mitchell SL, Kiley DK, Miller SC, et al. Hospice care for patients with dementia. J Pain Symptom Manage 2007;34:7–16.

4. Schonwetter RS, Han B, Small BJ, et al. Predictors of six-month survival among patients with dementia: an evaluation of hospice Medicare guidelines. Am J Hospice Palliative Care 2003;20:105–113.

5. Volicer L. End of life care for people with dementia in long-term care settings. Alzheimers Today 2008;9:84–102.

6. Mitchell SL, Kiely DK, Hamel MB. Dying with advanced dementia in the nursing home. Arch Intern Med 2004;164:321–326.

7. Kovach CR, Noonan PE, Schlidt AM, et al. A model of consequences of need-driven, dementia-compromised behavior. J Nurs Scholarship 2005;37:134–140.

8. Herr K, Coyne J, Key T, et al. Pain assessment in the nonverbal patient: Position statement with clinical practice recommendations. Pain Management Nurs 2006;7:44–52.

9. Kovach CR, Noonan PE, Griffie J, et al. The assessment of discomfort in dementia protocol. Pain Management Nurs 2002;3:16–27.

10. Schuler M, Njoo N, Hestermann M, et al. Acute and chronic pain in geriatrics: clinical characteristics of pain and the influence of cognition. Pain Med 2004;5:253–262.

11. Morrison RS, Siu AL. A comparison of pain and its treatment in advanced dementia and cognitively intact patients with hip fracture. J Pain Symptom Management 2000;19:240–248.

12. Etzioni S, Chodosh J, Ferrell BA, et al. Quality indicators for pain management in vulnerable elders. J Am Geriatr Soc 2007;55:S403–408.

13. Warden V, Hurley AC, Volicer L. Development and psychometric evaluation of the Pain Assessment in Advanced Dementia (PAINAD) scale. J Am Med Directors Assoc 2003;4:9–15.

14. Herr K, Decker S. Assessment of pain in older adults with severe cognitive impairment. Ann Long Term Care 2004;12:46–52.

15. Kovach CR, Noonan PE, Griffe J, et al. The assessment of discomfort in dementia protocol. Pain Management Nurs 2002;3:16–27.

16. Lefebre-Chaprio S. The Doloplus 2 scale: evaluating pain in the elderly. Eur J Palliative Care 2001;8:191–194.

17. Fuchs-Lacelle S, Hadjistavropoulos T. Development and preliminary validation of the pain Assessment Checklist for Seniors with Limited Ability to Communicate (PACSLAC). Pain Management Nurs 2004;5:37–49.

18. Snow A, Weber JB, O'Malley KJ, et al. NOPPAIN: a nursing assistant-administered pain assessment instrument for use in dementia. Dementia Geriatric Cognitive Disorders 2003;921:1–8.

19. American Geriatrics Society Panel on Persistent Pain in Older Persons. Clinical practice guideline: The management of persistent pain in older persons. J Am Geriatr Soc 2002;50:S205–224.

20. Manfredi P, Breuer B, Wallenstein S, et al. Opioid treatment for agitation in patients with advanced dementia. Int J Geriatr Psychiatry 2003;18:700–705.

21. Black BS, Finucane T, Baker A, et al. Health problems and correlates of pain in nursing home residents with advanced dementia. Alzheimers Dis Assoc Disorders 2006;20:283–290.

22. Wang SY, Fukagawa N, Hossain M, et al. Longitudinal weight changes, length of survival and energy requirements of long-term care residents with dementia. J Am Geriatr Soc 1997;45:1189–1195.

23. Mitchell SL. A 93-year-old man with advanced dementia and eating problems. JAMA 2007;298:2527–2536.

24. Volicer L. Medical issues in late-stage dementia. Alzheimers Care Quarterly 2005;6:29–34.

25. DiBartolo MC. Careful hand feeding: A reasonable alternative to PEG feeding in individuals with dementia. Nursing 2006;35:25–33.

26. Volicer L, Seltzer B. Rheaume Y. Eating difficulties in patients with probable dementia of the Alzheimer type. J Geriatr Psychiatry Neurol 1989;45:1002–1010.

27. Mitchell SL, Teno JM, Roy J, et al. A national study of the clinical and organizational determinants of tube-feeding among nursing home residents with advanced cognitive impairment. JAMA 2003;290:73–80.

28. Engel SE, Kiely DK, Mitchell SL. Satisfaction with end-of-life care from nursing home residents with advanced dementia. J Am Geriatr Soc 2006;54:1567–1572.

29. van der Steen JT, Ooms ME, van der Wal G, et al. Pneumonia: the demented patient's best friend? Discomfort after starting or withholding antibiotic treatment. J Am Geriatr Soc 2002;50:1681–1688.

30. D'Agata E, Mitchell SL. Patterns of antimicrobial use among nursing home residents with advanced dementia. Arch Intern Med 2008;168:357–362.

31. Holmes HM, Sach GA, Shega JW, et al. Integrating palliative medicine into care of persons with advanced dementia: Identifying appropriate medication use. J Am Geriatr Soc 2008;56:1306–1311.

32. Duthie EH. Medical care during late-stage dementia. In Kovach CR. Late-Stage Dementia Care: A Basic Guide. Taylor Francis, 1997.

33. Saliba D, Kington R, Buchanan J. Appropriateness of the decision to transfer nursing facility residents to the hospital. J Am Geriatr Soc 2000;48:154–163.

34. Hirschman KB, Joyce CM, James BD, et al. Do Alzheimer's disease patients want to participate in a treatment decision and would their caregivers let them? Gerontologist 2005;45:381–388.

35. Gjerdingen DK, Neff JA, Wang M, et al. Older persons' options about life-sustaining procedures in the face of dementia. Arch Fam Med 1999;8:954–958.

36. Mezey M, Kluger M, Maislin G, et al. Life-sustaining treatment decisions by spouses of patients with Alzheimer's disease. J Am Geriatr Soc 1996;44:144–150.

37. MacPhee E, Bickel K. Palliative care for patients with dementia: From diagnosis to bereavement. Ann Long Term Care 2007;15:41–47.

38. Meuser TM, Marwit SJ. A comprehensive, stage-sensitive model of grief in dementia caregiving. Gerontologist 2001;41:658–670.

39. Dougherty J, Gallagher M, Harrington P, et al. Joining the Journey: A Guide to Dementia Comfort Care. Hospice of the Valley, 2006.

40. Medical Guidelines for Determining Prognosis in Selected Non-Cancer Diseases. National Hospice and Palliative Care publication.

41. Miller SC, Mor V, Teno J. Hospice enrollment and pain assessment and management in nursing homes. J Pain Symptom Management 2003;26:791–799.

42. Schulz R, Belle SH, Czaja SJ, et al. Long-term care placement of dementia patients and caregiver health and well-being. JAMA 2004;292:961–967.

Chapter 18

Caring for the caregiver

AD caregivers are focused on the care, supervision, and quality of life of the patient with dementia. In parallel with disease progression, they are inexorably drawn into a vortex of the patient's ever-increasing needs, seemingly irrational and volatile behavior, withdrawal from society and family, declining communication, and self-absorption. The toll it extracts is enormous, yet both society and patients depend on the well-being of dementia caregivers.

Quantifying the "Burden" of Care

With more people living longer, the number of Americans with AD has doubled since 1980 to 4.5 million and is expected to triple again by 2050 (1). Seventy percent of patients are cared for at home (2), at a cost of care that averages $42,000 annually (3,4) and $174,000 over the lifetime of a dementia patient (5). There are an estimated 9.9 million unpaid caregivers in the United States; they are primarily family members (87%) but also include friends and neighbors (of all ages). In 2008, they provided 8.5 billion hours of unpaid care, a contribution to the nation valued at $94 billion (based on an average of the minimum wage and rates for nursing assistant care). Some patients have more than one unpaid caregiver—for example, people who live with their primary caregiver and also receive help from another relative, friend, or neighbor (6).

Limited amounts of care are covered by public programs; most is paid out of pocket by unpaid caregivers (6,7). This is a huge financial drain on families, but in cases where the patient and the caregiver spouse are still of employment age, it is even worse. In these instances, family and other unpaid caregivers must leave work or decrease their work hours, losing income and benefits, including employer contributions to their own retirement savings.

One third of caregivers have been providing care and support for at least 5 years and 39% from 1 to 4 years (6). In the United States, family caregivers save the government hundreds of millions of dollars by avoiding or postponing long-term care placement. It is, therefore, important from both governmental and personal perspectives to help caregivers stay healthy and find their roles satisfying and fulfilling. Most Americans want to care for family members, but they can seldom do it alone.

Job Description: Dementia Caregiver

Imagine what follows is a career description. Not many people would voluntarily pursue this path, yet as noted above many seem called to do so. A small subset are healthcare professionals, but the vast majority are laypeople whose loved one fell victim to AD, and they rose to the need to save their loved one. There are few better examples of noble human behavior. Typical caregiver duties across the disease continuum include:

Mild Dementia
- Recognize personality, memory, and other cognitive changes
- Acknowledge and discuss with patient
- Discuss with professional and seek formal diagnosis
- Make legal and financial plans
- Seek disease information
- Inform family
- Develop respite mechanisms
- Develop understanding of behavioral triggers
- Structure environment to enhance day-to-day function
- Modify communication techniques
- Support losses with direction and assistance
- Administer medications
- Provide emotional support to patient
- Supervise shopping
- Stop patient from driving
- Remove power tools, hazards
- Plan to inform friends
- Identify self as caregiver

Moderate Dementia
- The above responsibilities, plus:
- Re-evaluate transition of caregiver role ("Can I do this?" "Do I need help?" "What does the patient want?")
- Provide for increased personal care needs and deal with resistance to care
- Maintain responsibility for "patient story" and medical history
- Coordinate services, balanced with need to maintain patient's trust
- Deal with "cling"
- Provide constant cueing
- Develop activities and initiate
- Monitor for safety 24/7

- Watch for behavioral triggers
- Monitor patient's health and recognize disease progression
- Modify communication skills to prevent behavioral/aggressive outbursts
- Prevent wandering and develop a plan in case of elopement
- Administer all medications
- Communicate with patient, family, health providers
- Learn more about disease progression
- Begin to consider long-term care needs
- Evaluate care sites, begin to plan for placement or the next phase of care
- Care for own health
- Try to find ways to keep friends engaged and involved
- Find social support from both professionals and lay persons
- Function autonomously
- Grieve

Severe Dementia

- Provide all personal care, now including toileting, feeding, turning, and trying to prevent falls
- Manage urinary and fecal incontinence – often with patient resistance to protective products such as adult incontinence garments
- Skin care
- Evaluate for choking and difficulty with swallowing, modifying food consistency to minimize potential for aspiration
- Offer fluids frequently
- Identify weight loss and offer food frequently to increase caloric intake through high-fat calorie-dense foods and small frequent feedings.
- Identify and seek treatment for advancing complications, including sleep disorders, seizures, urinary tract infections, choking, pneumonias, contractures, and decubitus ulcers
- Seek emergency care for falls and sudden behavior changes
- Modify communication strategies
- Find "meaningful" activities, including adult day programming
- "To place or not to place": Find and help patient make the transition into long-term care and/or hospice care, and redefine the caregiver role
- Attend to staffing and oversee paid care (in many cases, daily)
- Translate and reinforce advance directives about feeding, antibiotic therapies, and hospitalizations
- Keep family informed
- Plan funeral arrangements
- Make plans to re-establish and reinvent self following patient death
- Grieve and "to let go and let God….." (8)

Caregivers often suffer from burden, guilt, fatigue, and depression as their responsibilities span years. Caregivers often neglect their own health, and some die during this period of prolonged stress. Caregiving stresses are compounded when caregivers must continue other responsibilities such as employment and raising children and grandchildren. Moreover, families are often conflicted about how caregiving should be accomplished or how much participation should be expected from each member (9,10). Caregiving responsibilities do not end even when the person with dementia is admitted to a care setting. Caregivers continue to monitor care, balance the expectations of themselves and other family members with the realities of long-term care environments, continue to provide some aspects of care, and advocate for their loved one.

Assessing Caregiver Status

Though it may seem self-evident, the first step in medically supporting a caregiver is to ensure the caregiver is your patient. Physicians should not be attempting to manage the health of patients whose medical history they do not know and whose medical records they cannot access. Often, the route to your office is led by the patient with dementia, not the caregiver. If the caregiver has a different physician than the dementia patient, these same principles apply, but communication between physicians must occur so that caregiver stresses observed by the dementia patient's doctor are communicated to the caregiver's doctor.

Depression

It is quite common for caregivers to become depressed during the course of the patient's illness. Caregivers often have a terrible time planning for their own needs. As the symptoms of their loved ones' illness become more pronounced and more demands are made on their time, caregivers often neglect social relationships and physical and emotional health. This experience can produce depression, anger, guilt, isolation, and physical illness. Moreover, friends and families may expect this degree of self-sacrifice as a part of the marriage vows or their perception of familial obligations. While some caregivers will complain, others will not recognize this in themselves. While discussing care of the patient, observe and listen for symptoms and observe for signs of depression (11). Caregiver depression also may be masked in caregiving jargon. The following are some signs of occult depression in caregivers:

- Sense of hopelessness in all activities ("Why bother taking him out? He won't remember anyway.")
- Fear of letting go of the patient by refusing services such as day care, a companion, or in-home respite services ("I know he would miss me and they couldn't meet his needs like I can")
- Taking the patient's mood-controlling medications, using alcohol, or combining alcohol with drugs ("The quetiapine doesn't help him much, but it sure helps me get a good night's sleep!")
- Neglecting own appearance ("I never have time to fix my hair any more")

- Neglecting own health, especially with statements expressing that death would be a release ("I've been out of my blood pressure medication for months")
- Allowing adult children or neighbors to dictate care decisions (My daughter [in another state] doesn't think it's time to place Mom.") </bl>

Depression, when present, should be treated, whether with antidepressants or another avenue. In more severe cases, formal psychiatric consultation should be sought.

Physical Problems

Even if the caregiver is not your patient, it is a good idea to know something about his or her health, assuming he or she has given you permission to obtain such information. Asking about the presence of chronic illnesses such as hypertension, heart disease, diabetes, cancer, and degenerative arthritis can provide an indicator of how much stress the caregiver can manage and when to press him or her to get help. Make note of bruises and skin tears, and ask about patient aggression toward the caregiver. As noted in the pharmacotherapy section, aggression is dangerous and can lead to serious caregiver injury. In such instances, better behavioral management for the patient should be sought, and this may necessitate a referral to a psychiatrist or neurologist or even inpatient management.

Helping the Caregiver: Services Available

Support Groups

Most people find support groups helpful because the participants share their situations, concerns, and sometimes remedies. The Alzheimer's Association Web site (www.alz.org) or chapter pamphlets can be used to locate the nearest group. It may take a few tries before the caregiver finds a group he or she likes, but it is well worth the effort. Some support groups offer services for the patient, such as respite while the caregiver attends the meeting and support groups for patients, and/or allow patients to attend with their caregiver. Sometimes special speakers visit and events are held. A support group can be an invaluable new resource to caregivers for making friends and social contacts. Events such as the Alzheimer's Association annual fundraiser "Memory Walk" can involve both patient and caregiver in positive social events that will reduce their sense of isolation and help both continue to feel engaged in the community. In some areas the Alzheimer's Association provides direct services with care coordinators. You need to check to see if the chapter in your area provides care management services and if they are provided by a licensed nurse or social worker. At times these services are provided by "trained volunteers," and the help offered varies enormously.

Telephone and In-Home Support Demonstrations

There have been several demonstration projects providing support to in-home caregivers (12–14) aimed at decreasing caregiver burden and depression. Telephone support was the most cost-effective way to provide such support. A demonstration project of telephone support by nurses at a home health agency led to improved caregiver satisfaction and use of community services, as well as reduced inpatient admissions and cost of care (13). Unfortunately, most such programs exist only for the term of a research grant.

On-Line Support Groups

For those who have access to a computer, there are numerous home pages and information sites for neurological diseases:

- Alzheimer's Association Message Board (http://www.alz.org/living_with_alzheimers_message_boards_lwa.asp): This is a forum for caregivers to ask questions and receive feedback from other caregivers and professionals, and for patients to receive support.
- Alzheimer List (http://alzheimer.wustl.edu/adrc2/alzheimerlist/): A valuable resource for people with memory loss, run by the Alzheimer's Disease Research Center at Washington University in St. Louis. This free site is accessed by sending an e-mail to mj2@lists.biostat.wustl.edu (Title: subscribe ALZHEIMER; Message: subscribe ALZHEIMER). Families will receive a confirmation notice with a phrase that must be copied and returned. Once that is done they will belong to a support group staffed by laypersons and professionals. They may simply read the e-mail messages or participate by sending or replying to messages. This support group is available 24/7 and is a great resource for practical answers on caregiving.

Internet Sites

There are numerous sites that provide information on AD and related disorders. As with anything on the World Wide Web, some sites are quite helpful while others may be filled with misinformation. Some helpful websites include the following:

- The Alzheimer's Association (http://www.alz.org): This is a comprehensive site developed to allow families and professionals to locate chapters of the Alzheimer's Association and resources nearest to them. The site also provides research updates and has a library of reference materials and caregiver information.
- National Institutes of Health, Clinical Trials Information (http://clinicaltrials.gov/): Families always want to ensure that the person with dementia is receiving the latest and best treatment available. This Web site provides information about medications currently being studied for AD, study sites, type of studies and their status, and whether the sites are recruiting subjects. To use the site, type "Alzheimer's disease" in the search box. If you are interested in participating in a study, type in "Alzheimer's disease" and the name of your city in the search box.

- NINDS Alzheimer's Disease Information Page (http://www.ninds.nih.gov/disorders/alzheimersdisease/alzheimersdisease.htm):
- Published by the U.S. Department of Health and Human Services, National Institute on Neurological Disorders and Stroke, this page provides up-to-date information on dementing illnesses and invaluable links to reputable organizations and information.
- National Institute on Aging ADEAR Center (http://www.nia.nih.gov/Alzheimers/).
- The Alzheimer's Disease Education and Referral (ADEAR) Center Web site will help you find current, comprehensive AD information and resources from the National Institute on Aging. One service offered by ADEAR is the Alzheimer's Fact Sheet (http://www.nia.nih.gov/Alzheimers/Publications/adfact.htm). This publication can be copied and distributed to friends and family who do not understand the basics of dementia.

Helping the Caregiver: Adult Children and Other Family Members

While caregivers come in a variety of relationships to the patient, the vast majority are spouses, and many such couples are elderly and have adult children to whom they may turn for help. Not all children, however, are comfortable in this situation. Common concerns of adult children include the following:

- "I don't want to remember Mom/Dad that way!"
- "I'm afraid." Some of the more common fears include the following:<sbl>
- Fear of violence
  - Fear of getting the disease
  - Fear of being rejected by the person with dementia, especially if asked to help with placement or removing the car
  - Fear of conflict with family members about how to provide care
  - Fear of being asked to provide more care than the adult child can handle
  - Fear that the caregiving experience might threaten a job or marriage
  - Fear of traumatizing grandchildren by exposing them to someone who is "not normal" or is frightening
  - Fear of the stigma of mental illness in the family

Adult children may have misconceptions and need to be counseled as to the meaning and implications of AD and dementia and what is needed for them to help. It is a good idea for the caregiver to voice the expectation that they will be needed to provide help, and even to generate a written list of needs to discuss (Table 18.1).

The caregiver must remember that often adult children need to be asked to help and then told how to help. You can help the caregiver to understand that this is an expectation for membership in the family. Family conflicts often emerge during this time. Each member will go through stages of grief at his or

Table 18.1 Ideas for Helping the Caregiver	
From a Distance	**Living Nearby**
Send funny greeting cards or flowers regularly.	Pick up dry cleaning.
Reviewing sources of information on the Internet and forwarding them	Take a casserole for dinner once a week.
Call at least twice a month and listen, even if it is repetitive or sad. Tell the caregiver and person with dementia how much you care.	Call or visit at least twice a month; when you visit, just listen.
Send news of your children and pictures.	Help with cleaning and fix-ups.
Plan to visit at least two or three times a year and stay in a hotel.	Take the person with dementia out for a meal.
Plan to attend diagnostic appointments.	Stay with the person while the caregiver gets a haircut.
Remember all birthdays, anniversaries, and holidays.	Serve as a sounding board without feeling like you have to "fix" problems.
Consult with other family members on specific needs.	Take the caregiver to a support group.
Send favorite foods occasionally.	Help to find local resources, including legal resources.
Send theater tickets or perhaps a subscription to a film rental service.	Monitor the person's driving.
Keep up to date on dementia for your family.	Help with legal and financial issues as appropriate.
Compliment the caregiver on a job well done, compliment nearby relatives on the help they provide.	Take the caregiver and person with dementia to church.
Plan to provide actual onsite respite once or twice a year for 1 or 2 days at a time.	Stay with the person so the caregiver can go to a favorite social group.

her own pace. Encourage the family to try to keep the arguments fair and seek help from a family therapist if needed.

Helping Caregivers to Take Care of Themselves

1. When talking with caregivers about the patient, it is often a good idea to suggest how the caregiver can also care for himself or herself:Eat a balanced diet.
2. Get adequate rest.
3. Drink plenty of fluids (1.5 to 2 quarts per day are suggested for good health).
4. Exercise at least three times a week (five is preferable) for a minimum of 20 minutes:
   (a) Walking, especially good if done with a friend

(b) Dancing with your loved one
(c) Gardening
(d) Bowling
(e) Swimming
(f) Mall-walking or shopping
(g) Exercising a pet
5. If you have symptoms of depression (see earlier in the chapter), consider treatment with an antidepressant.
6. Get annual health screenings.
7. Get flu and pneumonia vaccinations.
8. Make sure your tetanus immunization is current.
9. Get out with friends regularly.
10. Make sure you have some time alone each day.
11. Pursue a hobby, especially with family or friends.
12. Find something that makes you laugh and do it regularly.
13. Rent movies you enjoy.
14. Attend spiritual or religious services regularly.
15. Use respite services, especially adult day programming, as often as possible. With adult day programs, 3 days per week is recommended.
16. Attend support groups and keep in touch with helping professionals.
17. Do something challenging (crosswords or puzzles).
18. Splurge on yourself on a regular basis, whether clothing, a food treat, a long-distance phone call, or whatever makes you happy.

References

1. Hebert LE, Scherr PA, Bienias JL, et al. Alzheimer disease in the US population: prevalence estimates using the 2000 census. Arch Neurol 2003;60:1119–1122.

2. U.S.Congress Office of Technology Assessment. Losing a Million Minds: Confronting the Tragedy of Alzheimer's Disease and Other Dementias. U.S. Government Printing Office, 1987.

3. Rice DP, Fox PJ, Max W, et al. The economic burden of Alzheimer's disease care. Health Aff (Millwood) 1993;12:164–176.

4. Rice DP, Fillit HM, Max W, et al. Prevalence, costs, and treatment of Alzheimer's disease and related dementia: a managed care perspective. Am J Manag Care 2001;7:809–818.

5. Ernst RL, Hay JW. The US economic and social costs of Alzheimer's disease revisited. Am J Public Health 1994;84:1261–1264.

6. Alzheimer's Association. 2009 Alzheimer's facts and figures. Accessed April 16, 2009; available at: http://www.alz.org/national/documents/report_alzfactsfigures2009.pdf

7. Alzheimer's Association and National Alliance for Caregiving. Families Care: Alzheimer's Caregiving in the United States, 2004. Accessed April 13, 2009; available at: www.alz.org

8. Hall G. Mapping Dementia: Developmental Tasks along the Disease Trajectory. Iowa City: University of Iowa, 2000.

9. Whitlatch C. Informal caregivers: communication and decision making. Am J Nurs 2008;108(9 Suppl):73–77.

10. Cotter VT. The burden of dementia. Am J Managed Care 2007;13(Suppl 8): S193–197.

11. Connor KI, McNeese-Smith DK, Vickrey BG, et al. Determining care management activities associated with mastery and relationship strain for dementia caregivers. J Am Geriatr Soc 2008;56(5):891–897.

12. American Psychiatric Association. Diagnostic and Statistical Manual of Mental Disorders IV-TR, 4th ed, text revision. Washington DC: American Psychiatric Association, 2000.

13. Engelhardt J, Kiesiel T, Nicholson J, et al. Impact of a care coordination and support strategic partnership on clinical outcomes. Home Healthcare Nurse 2008;26(3):166–172.

14. Aupperle PM. Navigating patients and caregivers through the course of Alzheimer's disease. J Clin Psychiatry 2006;67(Suppl 3):8–14.

Experimental and future therapies

Recent advances in the understanding of AD pathophysiology have led to a surge in new treatments that are approaching or are already in clinical trials. The numbers are startling: there are five FDA-approved treatments for AD but *hundreds* in development. Clinicians need to have a sense of the kinds of therapies that may be on the horizon. Since the class or mechanism of action may be more useful to understand than the details of a specific agent, these emerging treatments will be presented according to the known or presumed (although in many cases not sole) pathophysiological process targeted by the particular therapy (Table E.1).

By definition, any organizing schematic is vulnerable to oversimplification, but the advantage of using this approach is that it affords a way to partially categorize a very large number of interventions. Those that are farthest along in development, or that best illustrate key trends in the field, will be described in more detail.

Table E.1 Categories of Experimental Therapies

Neurotransmitter-based therapies
- Acetylcholine
- Glutamate
- NMDA receptor
- AMPA receptor
- Histamine

Amyloid-modifying medications
- Active and passive amyloid-immunization therapies
- β-secretase inhibitors
- γ-secretase inhibitors
- Selective amyloid lowering agents (SALAs)
- Anti-aggregation therapies
- Cholesterol-lowering agents
- Metal chelators
- Curcumin
- PPAR-gamma agonists (insulin sensitizers)

Tau-phosphorylation inhibitors
- Glycogen synthase kinase inhibitors (e.g., lithium, valproate)

Antioxidants

Other
- Anti-inflammatory agents
- Anti-excitotoxic agents
- Neurotrophic agents
- Hormonal therapies

Chapter 19

Neurotransmitter-based interventions

Acetylcholine

AD patients have reduced production of choline acetyltransferase, a key enzyme in the synthesis of acetylcholine. This results in a decrease in acetylcholine synthesis and impaired cortical cholinergic function (1,2) as well as a reduction in cholinergic cell bodies in the nucleus basalis (2,3). Central cholinergic neurotransmission plays a critical role in cognition (4). Four cholinesterase inhibitors—tacrine, donepezil, rivastigmine, and galantamine—are FDA approved for use in AD (although tacrine is rarely if ever still used). Others in development include phenserine, huperzine A (isolated from Chinese club moss, *Huperzia serrata*), ZT-1 (a pro-drug of huperzine A), ladostigil, and bisnorcymserine (5).

There is a loss of nicotinic acetylcholine receptors (nAChRs) in the hippocampus and the temporal and frontal cortex in AD (6). In small studies, nicotine improved memory, cognition, and attention in patients with AD; nicotinic antagonists showed the opposite effect (7). Because nAChRs are found centrally and in the periphery, nicotine's utility has been limited by its peripheral effects. Selective CNS nicotinic agonists are in development, specifically targeting the $\alpha 4\beta 2$ subtype of nAChRs because of high densities of these receptors in brain regions involved in memory processes (6). Ispronicline (TC-1734) is a selective partial agonist at the central $\alpha 4\beta 2$ nAChRs that has shown positive effects on cognition in a double-blind, placebo-controlled crossover study of 76 subjects with age-associated memory impairment (8). The α-7 nAChR subtype has also received particular attention. There are several α-7 nicotinic agonists in development, including MEM 3454, SSR 180711C, PH-399733, and GTS-21 currently in phase II trials (5,9).

Glutamate

Glutamate is the primary excitatory amino acid in cortical and hippocampal neurons and plays an important role in synaptic transmission (10). Normally it binds to a variety of receptors, resulting in long-term potentiation of neuronal activity that may be critical in memory and learning. Excessive activation of receptors by glutamate destroys cells through what is termed excitotoxicity (11) and could impair cognition through impaired signal-to-noise ratio. It is possible that glutamatergic dysregulation plays a role in AD, and a variety of treatment approaches are based on this hypothesis.

NMDA Receptor Antagonists

N-methyl-D-aspartate (NMDA) receptor is one subtype of glutamate ionotropic receptor. Memantine is a noncompetitive NMDA receptor antagonist that decreases calcium ion influx under pathological conditions. Memantine received FDA approval for patients with moderate to severe AD in 2003, but not for patients with mild disease (12,13). Second-generation NMDA receptor antagonists, including delucemine and neramexane, are in development (5).

AMPA Receptor Modulators

The α-amino-3-hydroxy-5-methylisoxazole-4-propionic acid (AMPA) receptor, one of the main excitatory receptors in the CNS, is a non-NMDA-type ionotropic transmembrane glutamate receptor and is thought to play an important role in encoding memory through long-term potentiation (14–18). Ampakines are a class of drugs that augment ionic current flow through the AMPA receptor, enhancing fast, excitatory synaptic responses, and thus are thought to improve memory performance. A variety of ampakines have been developed, but none has shown significant benefit as yet (19).

Histamine

The H3 histamine receptor plays a role in control of arousal and cognition, suggesting that H3 receptor antagonists may improve cognition in AD (20). Several have been readied for clinical trials (21). One such drug, dimebon, is thought to block the histamine binding site of the NMDA receptor, thus modulating activity of NMDA receptors (22). It also inhibits acetylcholinesterase and may have other effects as well: proprietary data suggest that in fact non-neurotransmitter-based mechanisms involving mitochondrial function could account for dimebon's effects (23). Dimebon has been approved in Russia as an antihistamine since the early 1980s and is currently being investigated as a therapy for AD. A 6-month randomized, double-blind, placebo-controlled phase II trial in 183 patients with mild to moderate AD showed significant benefit on measures of cognition, global assessment, activities of daily living, global function, and behavior (24). Dimebon is in phase III development (25).

References

1. Bowen DM, Smith CB, White P, et al. Neurotransmitter-related enzymes and indices of hypoxia in senile dementia and other abiotrophies. Brain 1976;99(3):459–496.

2. Whitehouse PJ, Price DL, Struble RG, et al. Alzheimer's disease and senile dementia: loss of neurons in the basal forebrain. Science 1982;215(4537):1237–1239.

3. Arendt T, Bigl V, Arendt A, Tennstedt A. Loss of neurons in the nucleus basalis of Meynert in Alzheimer's disease, paralysis agitans and Korsakoff's disease. Acta Neuropathol 1983;61(2):101–108.

4. Bartus RT, Flicker C, Dean RL, et al. Behavioral and biochemical effects of nucleus basalis magnocellularis lesions: implications and possible relevance to understanding or treating Alzheimer's disease. Prog Brain Res 1986;70:345–361.

5. Pogacic V, Herrling P. List of drugs in development for neurodegenerative diseases. Update June 2007. Neurodegener Dis 2007;4(6):443–486.

6. Nordberg A. Nicotinic receptor abnormalities of Alzheimer's disease: therapeutic implications. Biol Psychiatry 2001;49(3):200–210.

7. Newhouse PA, Potter A, Kelton M, et al. Nicotinic treatment of Alzheimer's disease. Biol Psychiatry 2001;49(3):268–278.

8. Dunbar GC, Inglis F, Kuchibhatla R, et al. Effect of ispronicline, a neuronal nicotinic acetylcholine receptor partial agonist, in subjects with age-associated memory impairment (AAMI). J Psychopharmacol 2007;21(2):171–178.

9. Mazurov A, Hauser T, Miller CH. Selective alpha7 nicotinic acetylcholine receptor ligands. Curr Med Chem 2006;13(13):1567–1584.

10. Mattson MP, Pedersen WA, Duan W, et al. Cellular and molecular mechanisms underlying perturbed energy metabolism and neuronal degeneration in Alzheimer's and Parkinson's diseases. Ann N Y Acad Sci 1999;893:154–175.

11. Rothman SM, Thurston JH, Hauhart RE. Delayed neurotoxicity of excitatory amino acids in vitro. Neuroscience 1987;22(2):471–480.

12. Reisberg B, Doody R, Stoffler A, et al. Memantine in moderate-to-severe Alzheimer's disease. N Engl J Med 2003;348(14):1333–1341.

13. Tariot PN, Farlow MR, Grossberg GT, et al. Memantine treatment in patients with moderate to severe Alzheimer disease already receiving donepezil: a randomized controlled trial. JAMA 2004;291(3):317–324.

14. Staubli U, Perez Y, Xu FB, et al. Centrally active modulators of glutamate receptors facilitate the induction of long-term potentiation in vivo. Proc Natl Acad Sci U S A 1994;91(23):11158–11162.

15. Ingvar M, Ambros-Ingerson J, Davis M, et al. Enhancement by an ampakine of memory encoding in humans. Exp Neurol 1997;146(2):553–559.

16. Lynch G, Kessler M, Rogers G, et al. Psychological effects of a drug that facilitates brain AMPA receptors. Int Clin Psychopharmacol 1996;11(1):13–19.

17. Lynch G, Granger R, Imbros-Ingerson J, et al. Evidence that a positive modulator of AMPA-type glutamate receptors improves delayed recall in aged humans. Exp Neurol 1997;145(1):89–92.

18. Wezenberg E, Verkes RJ, Ruigt GS, et al. Acute effects of the ampakine farampator on memory and information processing in healthy elderly volunteers. Neuropsychopharmacology 2007;32(6):1272–1283.

19. Jhee SS, Chappell AS, Zarotsky V, et al. Multiple-dose plasma pharmacokinetic and safety study of LY450108 and LY451395 (AMPA receptor potentiators) and their concentration in cerebrospinal fluid in healthy human subjects. J Clin Pharmacol 2006;46(4):424–432.

20. Panula P, Rinne J, Kuokkanen K, et al. Neuronal histamine deficit in Alzheimer's disease. Neuroscience 1998;82(4):993–997.

21. Witkin JM, Nelson DL. Selective histamine H3 receptor antagonists for treatment of cognitive deficiencies and other disorders of the central nervous system. Pharmacol Ther 2004;103(1):1–20.

22. Grigorev VV, Dranyi OA, Bachurin SO. Comparative study of action mechanisms of dimebon and memantine on AMPA- and NMDA-subtypes glutamate receptors in rat cerebral neurons. Bull Exp Biol Med 2003;136(5):474–477.

23. www.medivation.com/pipeline_dimebon.html.

24. www.alzforum.org/new/detail.asp?id=1590.

25. www.medivation.com/pipeline_alzheimer.html.

Chapter 20

Amyloid-based interventions

Intervening with the amyloid cascade might decrease $A\beta_{42}$ production, reduce plaque formation, or decrease amyloid burden by increasing plaque clearance. Various anti-amyloid treatment agents are in or approaching clinical trials, as summarized here.

Immunotherapy

Immune activation might clear $A\beta$ from the brain through microglial-mediated phagocytosis, thus reducing $A\beta$ fibrils, oligomers, and/or amyloid plaque formation—or perhaps by creating a peripheral "sink" into which central amyloid species are cleared (1–3). Both active and passive immunization strategies are being studied. Active immunization involves introduction of the antigen, a variant of the $A\beta$ peptide, typically linked to an adjuvant, producing an immune response against that antigen in the host. Passive immunization involves delivery of synthetic antibodies against $A\beta$ peptide into the host, thereby facilitating immune-mediated clearance of the antigen. Both active and passive modes of immunization were found to be successful in clearing $A\beta$ deposits in transgenic mouse models of AD (4–9). Additionally, various cognitive deficits in transgenic models showed significant improvement with immunotherapy (10–12).

Active Immunotherapy

After success with $A\beta$ immunization in mouse models of AD, testing the same concept in patients began with AN1792, an aggregated human $A\beta_{42}$ peptide with Qs-21 adjuvant. This was the first active vaccine to be tested in humans. Phase I trials showed an adequate immune response without any serious adverse effects. A historic phase II clinical trial involving 300 people with mild to moderate AD was launched, but it was halted before completion when 6% of the participants treated with AN1792 developed a T-cell-based autoimmune meningoencephalitis (13). AN1792 immunization elicited excessive activation of T1 cells, leading to overactivation of inflammatory responses similar to those seen in autoimmune diseases (14).

Analyses of the accrued (though incomplete) clinical data showed no definite clinical benefit on primary outcome measures, although there was a suggestion of benefit on some secondary outcomes in the minority of patients who developed a significant antibody response (13). Among the small number of enrollees who subsequently died and went to autopsy, there was variable clearance of amyloid plaque burden among those who had received the active vaccine and achieved a significant antibody response (15), but serial MRIs showed an unexpected loss of brain volume among active vaccine recipients (16); even in these patients with neuropathological evidence of plaque clearing, dementia progression continued, apparently unabated (17).

These complexities notwithstanding, this study is viewed as having partially proved that amyloid pathology can be modified in patients with established AD. Current development efforts focus on activating highly specific antibody responses to $A\beta$, thus minimizing the adverse effects that were observed in the AN1792 phase II study. One example, ACC-001, is beginning phase II testing in patients with mild to moderate AD (18). Another, CAD106, consists of the first six N-terminal amino acids of $A\beta$ attached to a virus-like particle, which is believed to stimulate B cells while preventing excessive T-cell activation, thereby avoiding T-cell-mediated adverse effects (19). Other active vaccines nearing or already in clinical trials are proprietary (19).

Passive Immunotherapy

Passive immunization has advantages and disadvantages compared with active immunization. Less time is required by the host to generate an immune reaction. Active vaccination does not result in an adequate antibody response in all people, especially the elderly: this problem is moot with passive immunization. However, regular and frequent administration of antibodies is needed to carry on the immune-mediated clearance of the antigen by the host. There are also likely to be differences in safety and tolerability that remain to be shown, as well as differences in effectiveness.

Several different passive immunotherapy techniques are in development. The anti-$A\beta$ antibody, m266, has been found to restore cholinergic dysfunction and improve learning in APP transgenic mice (20). LY206430 is a humanized version of m266 that is in early clinical testing. AAB-001 (bapineuzumab) is a monoclonal antibody that is being studied in phase II clinical trials in about 200 patients with mild to moderate AD; phase III trials have been launched (21).

Human intravenous immunoglobulin (IVIg) is another approach. IVIg is already in use in the treatment of other neurological disorders and comes with the advantage of an established record of adverse effects. It apparently contains anti-$A\beta$ antibodies, and its administration has been found to increase the titer of anti-$A\beta$ antibodies in the blood (22). In vitro, anti-$A\beta$ antibodies from IVIg have been shown to disrupt $A\beta$ fibrillogenesis and exert neuroprotective effects (23). Open-label pilot studies with IVIg conducted by Dodel et al have shown 30% reduction in $A\beta$ in CSF, 233% increases in serum $A\beta$, and stabilization of ADAS-cog and MMSE scores (24). Another open-label study by Relkin et al reported similar findings with human IVIg (25). The first placebo-controlled trail is under way, and a phase III trial is being conducted by the Alzheimer's Disease Cooperative Study (26).

Secretase Inhibitors

β-secretase (β-site APP cleavage enzyme; BACE) and γ-secretase are enzymes that are involved in the pathological cleaving of the APP molecule, which results in the increased production of the toxic $A\beta_{42}$ peptide. Theoretically, interfering with their action has the potential to disrupt the amyloid cascade. BACE inhibitors probably represent the most attractive approach, as they target one of the initial events in the cascade. They are large molecules, making entry into the brain problematic. In addition, the receptor site is difficult to bind (3,27). No BACE inhibitor has survived beyond early clinical development (28).

γ-secretase cleaves a variety of substrates other than APP and controls many signaling systems involved in cell differentiation in embryogenesis and hematopoiesis (29,30). Therefore, inhibition of γ-secretase blocks not only the processing of APP but also other essential molecules such as the Notch signaling protein, which is an important intermediary in cellular functions like the regulation and differentiation of cells in the gastrointestinal tract and immune system (31,32). This action on Notch could result in untoward gastrointestinal and other adverse events. Current research in this area aims at finding compounds that are specific for γ-secretase cleavage of APP so that selective inhibition occurs only at that site.

LY450139 was the first functional γ-secretase inhibitor to be studied clinically, and initial studies showed marginal effects on CSF biomarkers in AD patients (33). Adverse effects included gastrointestinal toxicity, probably due to inhibition of Notch as well. More recent unpublished data, however, showed transient decreased production of Aβ species in humans: based largely on this finding, a phase III trial is under way (34). MK-0752 is a γ-secretase inhibitor that has been studied in a phase I clinical trial. Preliminary results have shown a reduction of CSF $A\beta_{40}$ levels, offering proof of concept; no serious adverse effects were observed (35). Other proprietary agents are in development.

Selective $A\beta_{42}$ Lowering Agents (SALAs)

This term refers to certain drugs that preferentially inhibit the formation of $A\beta_{42}$ over $A\beta_{40}$ and do not seem to affect the Notch system or inhibit γ-secretase (36,37). The first SALA to be studied clinically was R-flurbiprofen (tarenflurbil). It is a pure R-enantiomer of flurbiprofen and has the advantage of not possessing cyclooxygenase inhibitory effects, thus not carrying the burden of gastrointestinal or renal adverse effects associated with nonsteroidal anti-inflammatories (NSAIDs) (38). No benefit was seen on primary outcomes in a phase II trial in participants with mild to moderate AD, although a secondary analysis of patients with mild AD showed a significant improvement in cognition and function at the higher dosage. A 1-year open-label extension in patients with mild AD on higher dosages showed less decline than expected (39). Two phase III placebo-controlled trials of R-fluribuprofen in patients with mild AD showed no benefit (40).

Other nitric acid (NO)-releasing derivatives of flurbiprofen, HCT 1026 and NCX 2216, have shown anti-amyloidogenic activity in animal models (41). These compounds have the capacity to donate NO inside the cell, which is thought to improve the tolerability of the parent drug flurbiprofen (42). It remains to be seen whether these will be developed further.

Anti-Aggregation Agents

Aβ is normally present in the plasma and CSF in a soluble form, but under pathological conditions such as excessive production of Aβ, free radical damage, or unusually hydrophobic conditions, Aβ aggregates as oligomers, presumably beginning the toxic amyloid cascade (43–46). Several approaches are being studied to inhibit Aβ aggregation.

Tramiprosate, a drug that acts as an amyloid antagonist, interferes with the amyloid cascade by binding to the soluble Aβ peptide, thus preventing the downstream toxic effects of Aβ deposition. In animal studies it produced a dose-dependent decrease in both soluble and insoluble Aβ_{40} and Aβ_{42} levels. A phase II study with patients with mild to moderate AD over 3 months showed no effect on cognition after 3 months, and a dose-dependent reduction in CSF Aβ_{42} levels but not Aβ_{40} was observed after 3 months (47). This led to a multicenter phase III trial of 1,050 patients that failed to show efficacy; the second phase III trial has been halted (48).

Fibril formation due to aggregation of Aβ is strongly facilitated by phosphatidyl-inositolipids. Scyllo-cyclohexanehexol (AZD-103) is a phosphatidyl-inositolipid derivative that competes with phophatidyl-inositolipids for Aβ binding, thereby interfering with Aβ fibril formation. After an initial phase I study proved its tolerability, further development has been announced (49). This agent is of considerable interest by virtue of its mechanism of action as well as its promise of good tolerability and safety.

Statins

Epidemiological studies have suggested an association between cholesterol-lowering therapy with HMG-CoA reductase inhibitors and a lower risk of AD (50,51). Animal models have shown that decreasing cholesterol was associated with decreased amyloid deposition in the brain. It was also observed that increased dietary cholesterol increased brain amyloid in animals. The mechanism is thought to be through reduced inflammation with cholesterol reduction as well as enhanced α-secretase activity by statins. Activating the α-secretase pathway shifts Aβ processing away from β-secretase and γ-secretase, decreasing production of the toxic $A\beta_{42}$.

In a small randomized placebo-controlled study, simvastatin showed a decrease in $A\beta_{40}$ in a post hoc analysis of a subgroup with mild AD but did not show significant alteration in CSF levels of Aβ overall (52). Another randomized placebo-controlled trial of atorvastatin in 67 patients with mild to moderate AD over 12 months did not show statistically significant benefit (53). Two other phase III placebo-controlled studies with simvastatin and atorvastatin have been completed and have been reported to show negative results (54).

Metal Chelators

Heavy metal ions are thought to play a role in fibrillization of Aβ; therefore, heavy metal chelators may reduce polymerization. Clioquinol, a drug with copper and zinc chelation properties, has shown to reduce brain amyloid in transgenic mouse models of AD (55). A phase II study in 36 patients with moderate to severe AD showed a decline in plasma Aβ levels but failed to show any cognitive benefit (56). Clioquinol was used in the past for parasitic gastrointestinal disease but was associated with a rare form of optic nerve damage called subacute myelo-opticoneuropathy (57). Further development of this drug has been halted due to concerns regarding toxicity and impurities in the formulation. PBT-2 is a clioquinol analogue that has completed a phase IIa study with 78 patients over 12 weeks; it was safe and well tolerated, showing encouraging cognitive effects (58).

Curcumin

Curcumin is the active ingredient in turmeric powder, which has shown to possess antioxidant and disaggregation properties. It has been shown to reduce oxidative damage in a transgenic mouse model of AD (59), inhibit $A\beta_{40}$ aggregation in a dose-dependent manner in vitro (60), and inhibit oligomerization and fibril formation and reduce amyloid burden in vivo (61). However, curcumin showed no benefit in a small clinical trial (62).

Peroxisome Proliferator-Activated Receptor-γ Agonists

Insulin resistance induces chronic peripheral insulin elevations and reduces brain insulin levels. Many theories of how insulin influences AD pathophysiology have been proposed. Chief among them is the fact that Aβ is a substrate for insulin degrading enzyme (IDE); if insulin levels are chronically elevated, it is possible that Aβ degradation would be impaired. Insulin modulates glucose utilization in selective CNS circuits, which could affect cognition. Insulin is also thought to affect neurotransmitter levels (63). It may also contribute to cerebral inflammation (64).

Peroxisome proliferator-activated receptor-γ (PPAR-γ) agonists improve insulin sensitivity. A pilot study by Watson et al showed improvement in delayed recall (65). A trial of 511 nondiabetic AD patients over 6 months did not show significant effects, but a secondary analysis found that subjects without the APOE ε4 allele showed improvements compared to placebo (66). Three multicenter placebo-controlled trials are under way to assess rosiglitazone in AD patients stratified by APOE status to further study this possible effect (67).

Docosahexaenoic Acid (DHA)

Epidemiological studies suggest a reduced risk of developing AD associated with fish consumption (68,69). Docosahexaenoic acid (DHA) is one of the major omega-3 fatty acids found in fish oil and is an integral component of neural membrane phospholipids and the major polyunsaturated fatty acid in the brain (70). Animal studies support using DHA as treatment for AD by means of anti-amyloid, antioxidant, and neuroprotective mechanisms. Safety and tolerability studies (71) have led the way to a large multicenter phase III randomized placebo-controlled study being conducted by the Alzheimer's Disease Cooperative Study (72).

References

1. Gelinas DS, DaSilva K, Fenili D, et al. Immunotherapy for Alzheimer's disease. Proc Natl Acad Sci USA 2004;101(Suppl 2):14657–14662.

2. Tariot PN. Clinical trials of amyloid-based therapies for Alzheimer's disease. CNS Spectr 2007;12(1 Suppl 1):7–10.

3. Walker LC, Ibegbu CC, Todd CW, et al. Emerging prospects for the disease-modifying treatment of Alzheimer's disease. Biochem Pharmacol 2005;69(7):1001–1008.

4. Schenk D, Barbour R, Dunn W, et al. Immunization with amyloid-beta attenuates Alzheimer-disease-like pathology in the PDAPP mouse. Nature 1999;400(6740):173–177.

5. Janus C, Pearson J, McLaurin J, et al. A beta peptide immunization reduces behavioural impairment and plaques in a model of Alzheimer's disease. Nature 2000;408(6815):979–982.

6. Sigurdsson EM, Scholtzova H, Mehta PD, et al. Immunization with a nontoxic/nonfibrillar amyloid-beta homologous peptide reduces Alzheimer's disease-associated pathology in transgenic mice. Am J Pathol 2001;159(2):439–447.

7. Bard F, Cannon C, Barbour R, et al. Peripherally administered antibodies against amyloid beta-peptide enter the central nervous system and reduce pathology in a mouse model of Alzheimer disease. Nat Med 2000;6(8):916–919.

8. Lombardo JA, Stern EA, McLellan ME, et al. Amyloid-beta antibody treatment leads to rapid normalization of plaque-induced neuritic alterations. J Neurosci 2003;23(34):10879–10883.

9. Wilcock DM, DiCarlo G, Henderson D, et al. Intracranially administered anti-Abeta antibodies reduce beta-amyloid deposition by mechanisms both independent of and associated with microglial activation. J Neurosci 2003;23(9):3745–3751.

10. Morgan D, Diamond DM, Gottschall PE, et al. A beta peptide vaccination prevents memory loss in an animal model of Alzheimer's disease. Nature 2000;408(6815):982–985.

11. Kotilinek LA, Bacskai B, Westerman M, et al. Reversible memory loss in a mouse transgenic model of Alzheimer's disease. J Neurosci 2002;22(15):6331–6335.

12. Lee EB, Leng LZ, Zhang B, et al. Targeting amyloid-beta peptide (Abeta) oligomers by passive immunization with a conformation-selective monoclonal antibody improves learning and memory in Abeta precursor protein (APP) transgenic mice. J Biol Chem 2006;281(7):4292–4299.

13. Gilman S, Koller M, Black RS, et al. Clinical effects of Abeta immunization (AN1792) in patients with AD in an interrupted trial. Neurology 2005;64(9):1553–1562.

14. Orgogozo JM, Gilman S, Dartigues JF, et al. Subacute meningoencephalitis in a subset of patients with AD after Abeta42 immunization. Neurology 2003;61(1):46–54.

15. Nicoll JA, Wilkinson D, Holmes C, et al. Neuropathology of human Alzheimer disease after immunization with amyloid-beta peptide: a case report. Nat Med 2003;9(4):448–452.

16. Orgogozo JM. Vaccination treatment of AD (abstract S5–04-04). Alzheimers Dementia 2006;2(3):S94.

17. Holmes C, Boche D, Wilkinson D, et al. Long-term effects of Abeta42 immunisation in Alzheimer's disease: follow-up of a randomised, placebo-controlled phase I trial. Lancet 2008;372:216–223.

18. www.clinicaltrials.gov/ct2/show/NCT00479557?term=acc-001&rank=1

19. Woodhouse A, Dickson TC, Vickers JC. Vaccination strategies for Alzheimer's disease: A new hope? Drugs Aging 2007;24(2):107–119.

20. Bales KR, Tzavara ET, Wu S, et al. Cholinergic dysfunction in a mouse model of Alzheimer disease is reversed by an anti-A beta antibody. J Clin Invest 2006;116(3):825–832.

21. www.elan.com/news/2007/20070521.asp

22. Dodel RC, Hampel H, Du Y. Immunotherapy for Alzheimer's disease. Lancet Neurol 2003;2(4):215–220.

23. Du Y, Wei X, Dodel R, et al. Human anti-beta-amyloid antibodies block beta-amyloid fibril formation and prevent beta-amyloid-induced neurotoxicity. Brain 2003;126(Pt 9):1935–1939.

24. Dodel RC, Du Y, Depboylu C, et al. Intravenous immunoglobulins containing antibodies against beta-amyloid for the treatment of Alzheimer's disease. J Neurol Neurosurg Psychiatry 2004;75(10):1472–1474.

25. Relkin NR, Szabo P, Adamiak B, et al. 18-month study of intravenous immunoglobulin for treatment of mild Alzheimer disease. Neurobiol Aging 2008 Feb 20 [Epub].

26. www.baxter.com/about_baxter/news_room/news_releases/2007/08–28-07-ivig.html

27. Citron M. Strategies for disease modification in Alzheimer's disease. Nat Rev Neurosci 2004;5(9):677–685.

28. Hills ID, Vacca JP. Progress toward a practical BACE-1 inhibitor. Curr Opin Drug Discov Devel 2007;10(4):383–391.

29. Evin G, Sernee MF, Masters CL. Inhibition of gamma-secretase as a therapeutic intervention for Alzheimer's disease: prospects, limitations and strategies. CNS Drugs 2006;20(5):351–372.

30. Selkoe DJ, Schenk D. Alzheimer's disease: molecular understanding predicts amyloid-based therapeutics. Annu Rev Pharmacol Toxicol 2003;43:545–584.

31. Pollack SJ, Lewis H. Secretase inhibitors for Alzheimer's disease: challenges of a promiscuous protease. Curr Opin Investig Drugs 2005;6(1):35–47.

32. Wong GT, Manfra D, Poulet FM, et al. Chronic treatment with the gamma-secretase inhibitor LY-411,575 inhibits beta-amyloid peptide production and alters lymphopoiesis and intestinal cell differentiation. J Biol Chem 2004;279(13):12876–12882.

33. Siemers E, Skinner M, Dean RA, et al. Safety, tolerability, and changes in amyloid beta concentrations after administration of a gamma-secretase inhibitor in volunteers. Clin Neuropharmacol 2005;28(3):126–132.

34. www.newsroom.lilly.com/ReleaseDetail.cfm?ReleaseID=302104

35. Rosen LB, Stone J, Plump A, et al. The gamma secretase inhibitor MK-0752 acutely and significantly reduces CSF Abeta40 concentrations in humans. Alzheimers Dementia 2006;2(3):S79.

36. Beher D, Clarke EE, Wrigley JD, et al. Selected non-steroidal anti-inflammatory drugs and their derivatives target gamma-secretase at a novel site. Evidence for an allosteric mechanism. J Biol Chem 2004;279(42):43419–43426.

37. Weggen S, Eriksen JL, Sagi SA, et al. Abeta42-lowering nonsteroidal anti-inflammatory drugs preserve intramembrane cleavage of the amyloid precursor protein (APP) and ErbB-4 receptor and signaling through the APP intracellular domain. J Biol Chem 2003;278(33):30748–30754.

38. Townsend KP, Pratico D. Novel therapeutic opportunities for Alzheimer's disease: focus on nonsteroidal anti-inflammatory drugs. FASEB J 2005;19(12):1592–1601.

39. Wilcock G, Black S, Haworth J, et al. A placebo-controlled, double-blind trial of the selective Abeta-42 lowering agent, flurizan (MPC-7869, (R)-flurbiprofen) in patients with mild to moderate Alzheimer's disease. Alzheimers Dementia 2005;1(1, Suppl):S95.

40. www.myriad.com/alzheimers/flurizan.php

41. Gasparini L, Ongini E, Wilcock D, et al. Activity of flurbiprofen and chemically related anti-inflammatory drugs in models of Alzheimer's disease. Brain Res Brain Res Rev 2005;48(2):400–408.

42. Wallace JL, Muscara MN, de NG, et al. Gastric tolerability and prolonged prostaglandin inhibition in the brain with a nitric oxide-releasing flurbiprofen derivative, NCX-2216 [3-[4-(2-fluoro-alpha-methyl-[1,1'-biphenyl]-4-acetyloxy)-3-methoxyphenyl]-2-propenoic acid 4-nitrooxy butyl ester]. J Pharmacol Exp Ther 2004;309(2):626–633.

43. Seubert P, Vigo-Pelfrey C, Esch F, et al. Isolation and quantification of soluble Alzheimer's beta-peptide from biological fluids. Nature 1992;359(6393):325–327.

44. Shoji M, Golde TE, Ghiso J, et al. Production of the Alzheimer amyloid beta protein by normal proteolytic processing. Science 1992;258(5079):126–129.

45. Caughey B, Lansbury PT. Protofibrils, pores, fibrils, and neurodegeneration: separating the responsible protein aggregates from the innocent bystanders. Annu Rev Neurosci 2003;26:267–298.

46. Hull M, Berger M, Heneka M. Disease-modifying therapies in Alzheimer's disease: how far have we come? Drugs 2006;66(16):2075–2093.

47. Aisen PS, Saumier D, Briand R, et al. A phase II study targeting amyloid-beta with 3APS in mild-to-moderate Alzheimer disease. Neurology 2006;67(10):1757–1763.

48. www.alzforum.org/drg/drc/detail.asp?id=84

49. www.transitiontherapeutics.com/technology/alzheimers.php

50. Jick H, Zornberg GL, Jick SS, et al. Statins and the risk of dementia. Lancet 2000;356(9242):1627–1631.

51. Wolozin B, Kellman W, Ruosseau P, et al. Decreased prevalence of Alzheimer disease associated with 3-hydroxy-3-methyglutaryl coenzyme A reductase inhibitors. Arch Neurol 2000;57(10):1439–1443.

52. Simons M, Schwarzler F, Lutjohann D, et al. Treatment with simvastatin in normocholesterolemic patients with Alzheimer's disease: A 26-week randomized, placebo-controlled, double-blind trial. Ann Neurol 2002;52(3):346–350.

53. Sparks DL, Sabbagh MN, Connor DJ, et al. Atorvastatin for the treatment of mild to moderate Alzheimer disease: preliminary results. Arch Neurol 2005;62(5):753–757.

54. Kivipelto M, Solomon A, Winblad B. Statin therapy in Alzheimer's disease. Lancet Neurol 2005;4(9):521–522.

55. Cherny RA, Atwood CS, Xilinas ME, et al. Treatment with a copper-zinc chelator markedly and rapidly inhibits beta-amyloid accumulation in Alzheimer's disease transgenic mice. Neuron 2001;30(3):665–676.

56. Ritchie CW, Bush AI, Mackinnon A, et al. Metal-protein attenuation with iodochlorhydroxyquin (clioquinol) targeting Abeta amyloid deposition and toxicity in Alzheimer disease: a pilot phase 2 clinical trial. Arch Neurol 2003;60(12):1685–1691.

57. Tateishi J. Subacute myelo-optico-neuropathy: clioquinol intoxication in humans and animals. Neuropathology 2000;20(Suppl):S20–S24.

58. www.pranabio.com

59. Lim GP, Chu T, Yang F, et al. The curry spice curcumin reduces oxidative damage and amyloid pathology in an Alzheimer transgenic mouse. J Neurosci 2001;21(21):8370–8377.

60. Ono K, Hasegawa K, Naiki H, et al. Curcumin has potent anti-amyloidogenic effects for Alzheimer's beta-amyloid fibrils in vitro. J Neurosci Res 2004;75(6):742–750.

61. Yang F, Lim GP, Begum AN, et al. Curcumin inhibits formation of amyloid beta oligomers and fibrils, binds plaques, and reduces amyloid in vivo. J Biol Chem 2005;280(7):5892–5901.

62. clinicaltrials.gov/ct2/show/NCT00099710?term=curcumin&rank=8

63. Craft S. Insulin resistance syndrome and Alzheimer disease: pathophysiologic mechanisms and therapeutic implications. Alzheimer Dis Assoc Disord 2006;20(4):298–301.

64. Hak AE, Pols HA, Stehouwer CD, et al. Markers of inflammation and cellular adhesion molecules in relation to insulin resistance in nondiabetic elderly: the Rotterdam study. J Clin Endocrinol Metab 2001;86(9):4398–4405.

65. Watson GS, Cholerton BA, Reger MA, et al. Preserved cognition in patients with early Alzheimer disease and amnestic mild cognitive impairment during treatment with rosiglitazone: a preliminary study. Am J Geriatr Psychiatry 2005;13(11):950–958.

66. Risner ME, Saunders AM, Altman JF, et al. Efficacy of rosiglitazone in a genetically defined population with mild-to-moderate Alzheimer's disease. Pharmacogenomics J 2006;6(4):246–254.

67. www.alzforum.org/drg/drc/detail.asp?id=116

68. Kalmijn S, Launer LJ, Ott A, et al. Dietary fat intake and the risk of incident dementia in the Rotterdam Study. Ann Neurol 1997;42(5):776–782.

69. Barberger-Gateau P, Letenneur L, Deschamps V, et al. Fish, meat, and risk of dementia: cohort study. BMJ 2002;325(7370):932–933.

70. Lauritzen L, Hansen HS, Jorgensen MH, et al. The essentiality of long chain omega-3 fatty acids in relation to development and function of the brain and retina. Prog Lipid Res 2001;40(1–2):1–94.

71. Arterburn LM, Hall EB, Oken H. Distribution, interconversion, and dose response of omega-3 fatty acids in humans. Am J Clin Nutr 2006;83(6 Suppl):1467S–1476S.

72. www.clinicaltrials.gov/ct/show/NCT00440050

Chapter 21

Tau-based interventions

Tau, a protein widely expressed in the CNS, is encoded for by the microtubule-associated protein tau gene (1). Hyperphosphorylation of tau protein causes destabilization of microtubules and the pathological tau protein then clumps together to form neurofibrillary tangles, resulting in neuronal dysfunction. Normally only two or three residues on tau bear phosphates, but in AD and other tauopathies, this number can be up to nine (2). Hyperphosphorylation is associated with an imbalance in the activity levels of tau kinases and phosphatases (3). Inhibition of tau hyperphosphorylation is being pursued as a viable strategy for AD treatment through inhibitors of the three main kinases—GSK3β (glycogen synthase kinase 3β), CDK5 (cyclin-dependent kinase 5), and ERK2 (extracellular signal-regulated kinase 2) (4). Inhibition of microtubule-affinity-regulating kinase (MARK) is also being targeted as a possible strategy for intervention in AD (4). Comparable to the findings on amyloid plaques, some investigators believe that abnormal tau is the toxic agent and not neurofibrillary tangles (5,6). This area of clinical development lags far behind that for amyloid-based therapies. A few clinical trials have been launched; none has shown definitive results.

Valproate and lithium are being studied as possible AD therapies, partly based on preclinical and basic studies suggesting that they have anti-amyloid and neuroprotective properties (7). Glycogen synthase kinases (GSK)-3alpha/beta also play an important role in the phosphorylation of tau. Valproate appears to be an indirect inhibitor of GSK-3 and may protect against cell damage due to endoplasmic reticulum stress (8). A multicenter phase III clinical trial is under way assessing the potential neuroprotective effects of valproate in AD patients (7). Lithium is also known to inhibit GSK-3; however, a phase II trial was negative (9,10).

References

1. Binder LI, Frankfurter A, Rebhun LI. The distribution of tau in the mammalian central nervous system. J Cell Biol 1985;101(4):1371–1378.

2. Stoothoff WH, Johnson GV. Tau phosphorylation: physiological and pathological consequences. Biochim Biophys Acta 2005;1739(2–3):280–297.

3. Churcher I. Tau therapeutic strategies for the treatment of Alzheimer's disease. Curr Top Med Chem 2006;6(6):579–595.

4. Mazanetz MP, Fischer PM. Untangling tau hyperphosphorylation in drug design for neurodegenerative diseases. Nat Rev Drug Discov 2007;6(6):464–479.

5. Tanzi RE. Tangles and neurodegenerative disease—a surprising twist. N Engl J Med 2005;353(17):1853–1855.

6. SantaCruz K, Lewis J, Spires T, et al. Tau suppression in a neurodegenerative mouse model improves memory function. Science 2005;309(5733):476–481.

7. Tariot PN, Loy R, Ryan JM, et al. Mood stabilizers in Alzheimer's disease: symptomatic and neuroprotective rationales. Adv Drug Deliv Rev 2002;54(12):1567–1577.

8. Kim AJ, Shi Y, Austin RC, et al. Valproate protects cells from ER stress-induced lipid accumulation and apoptosis by inhibiting glycogen synthase kinase-3. J Cell Sci 2005;118(Pt 1):89–99.

9. www.nia.nih.gov/Alzheimers/ResearchInformation/NewsReleases/Archives/PR2006/PR20061017ADCS.htm

10. Hampel H, Ewers M, Burger K, et al. Lithium trial in Alzheimer's disease: A randomized, single-blind, placebo-controlled, multicenter 10 week study. J Clin Psychiatry 2009;70:922–931.

Chapter 22

Other agents

Antioxidants

Oxidative stress and free radicals play an important role in AD pathogenesis (1). A variety of antioxidants have been studied for AD treatment.

Selegiline has antioxidant as well as other relevant mechanisms of action: it is a monoamine oxidase-B (MAO-B) inhibitor that increases brain levels of dopamine and some trace neurotransmitters such as phenylethylamine, without affecting norepinephrine levels. It is currently marketed for the treatment of Parkinson's disease. Selegiline may have neuroprotective properties. Numerous clinical trials with selegiline in AD treatment have been performed, with variable results and insufficient evidence to justify routine clinical use (2). A comparison of vitamin E and selegiline in outpatients with moderate to severe dementia (3) found both drugs to have a small effect. A subsequent trial in MCI patients comparing vitamin E with donepezil and placebo did not find significant benefit of vitamin E (4).

Ginkgo biloba extract is thought to exert neuroprotective effects under conditions of hypoxia-ischemia, preventing neuronal cell death, inhibiting the toxic effects of Aβ, and acting as a free radical scavenger. However, the most recent study, a 6-month placebo-controlled trial involving over 500 patients with mild to moderate AD, showed no impact (5). A long-term prevention trial involving over 2,500 patients followed over 3 years for the development of dementia was also negative (6).

Anti-Inflammatory Medications

Epidemiological evidence supports the use of nonsteroidal anti-inflammatories as AD prophylaxis, but clinical trials data are negative. Low-dose prednisone (10 mg) did not prove effective in a 1-year-long, placebo-controlled trial by the Alzheimer's Disease Cooperative Study (7). There have been clinical trials failures with the cyclooxygenase-2 inhibitors celecoxib and rofecoxib, as well as with the nonspecific cyclooxygenase inhibitor naproxen (8). In addition, neither celecoxib nor naproxen showed significant cognitive benefit in a large prevention trial (9). Thus, the overall efficacy of anti-inflammatory agents in AD has yet to be demonstrated.

Anti-Excitotoxic Therapies

An increase in intracellular free calcium is thought to activate destructive enzymes like proteases, endonucleases, and phospholipases that contribute to neuronal death in the aging process and AD. Blocking the increase in intracellular free calcium might therefore slow disease progression. Nimodipine is a calcium channel blocker that has shown benefits in some AD clinical trials (10), but a meta-analysis of dementia trials concluded that there was no justification for long-term use (11). MEM 1003, another calcium channel blocker, has a longer elimination half-life than nimodipine and does not appear to affect blood pressure significantly. A phase II study in patients with mild to moderate AD was recently concluded without demonstrating benefit (12).

Neurotrophic Factors

Nerve growth factor (NGF), a trophic factor for cholinergic neurons, may target forebrain cholinergic neurons that release the majority of acetylcholine in the cortex and hippocampus. Degeneration of this cell population may contribute to cognitive decline in AD. NGF does not cross the blood–brain barrier, so delivering it to the brain has been a challenge. Investigators have introduced the NGF gene into the CNS by engineering the patient's own fibroblasts to produce human NGF, and then stereotactically injecting the cells into the nucleus basalis (13). There were some complications resulting from the procedure, but six patients without surgical complications were followed for 18 to 24 months. Compared to historical controls, rates of cognitive decline appeared to be slowed. Brain autopsy in one patient who died showed survival of the implanted autologous fibroblasts with little evidence of inflammation. This trial serves as an impetus for future studies in gene therapy. A new gene delivery method using adeno-associated virus is completing a phase I trial, and a phase II trial is in the planning stages (14).

A variety of other neurotrophic agents have been studied, mostly with disappointing results (15–17).

Estrogen

Estrogens may have cholinergic neurotrophic and neuroprotective effects and may enhance cognitive function (18). A beneficial role for estrogen in AD, cognitive function, mood, and aging is suggested by observations of an inverse relationship of estrogen replacement therapy dose and duration with dementia diagnoses on death certificates (19) and by preliminary trials suggesting cognitive-enhancing effects of estradiol, estrone, and conjugated estrogens in AD (20,21). The vast majority of postmenopausal women do not receive estrogen replacement therapy, spending the last third of their lives in an estrogen-deficient state, a time during which the risk of AD exponentially increases.

Unfortunately, clinical trials of conjugated equine estrogens to improve cognition in both hysterectomized and nonhysterectomized women with AD have not led to success, and indeed subjects fared somewhat worse both in cognition and safety; for instance, 5% developed deep vein thrombosis (22–24). The Women's Health Initiative Memory Study (WHIMS), a randomized, double-blind, placebo-controlled clinical trial, examined whether postmenopausal estrogen supplementation (both estrogen alone and estrogen plus progestin) reduces the risk of all-cause dementia (primary outcome) and subclinical (mild) cognitive impairment (secondary outcome) in healthy women aged 65 years or older (25). The estrogen-plus-progestin group was discontinued prematurely because women in this intervention group were at increased risk for heart disease, stroke, pulmonary embolism, and breast cancer compared with women receiving placebo. Furthermore, estrogen-plus-progestin therapy increased the risk for probable dementia in postmenopausal women aged 65 years or older and did not prevent MCI.

Conclusion

Meaningful advances in the understanding of the evolution of AD have led to discovery and preclinical development of many targets for development, based on vastly different foundations. A major unknown is whether data from cell and animal models will translate to clinical development success; the extent to which this is the case could have a major impact on future development approaches.

Neurotransmitter-based therapies have the potential to improve cognition and/or alter the pathobiology of AD. At present, it appears that amyloid-based therapies are the farthest along in development, and results suggest that amyloid dysregulation can be interrupted. It is unknown, however, whether this will actually yield clinical benefit.

Tangle burden correlates most closely with severity of cognitive impairment. Antitangle therapies are early in development, and it will be some time before we can establish proof of concept clinically. As this brief review suggests, there are hundreds of agents in the pipeline. Successful completion of large numbers of clinical trials may be the rate-limiting step to finding new treatments, so we need to find creative ways to accelerate the development of promising candidates. There are several options. Given that many new interventions target specific pathways that can be measured biologically, the opportunity exists to capitalize on spinal fluid, blood, and possibly urine biomarkers in smaller, rapid, go/no go proof-of-concept studies early in the clinical development process. Further, emerging imaging techniques exist for assessing structure, neuronal function, and molecular pathology, holding promise that these kinds of outcomes can also be used as therapeutic surrogates. Results from the Alzheimer's Disease Neuroimaging Initiative, a multicenter longitudinal study incorporating imaging, biomarker, and clinical outcomes in various clinical groups, will prove critical as we learn how biological and imaging markers change over time and how they relate to evolving clinical phenotype. These data will serve as a critical benchmark against which to measure emerging therapeutic surrogates. Enrichment techniques may prove useful as well, such as incorporating genetic information in participant selection in highly selected studies. A potential threat may be a shortage of sophisticated clinical investigators, particularly with the capability of deploying increasingly sophisticated imaging and other biomarker techniques, as well as of research participants.

The field must also be prepared to transform its approach to prevention as well, for instance by using imaging techniques to track Alzheimer's-like brain changes in healthy people carrying common susceptibility genes. These markers of disease evolution could be studied in proof-of-principle studies of risk-reducing or even prevention therapies without having to enroll thousands of subjects and waiting decades for results.

We are faced with a panoply of promising interventions. Some of these targets hold promise for treatment of those affected, some may have potential for prevention, some for both. It is too soon to predict which, if any, of these approaches will bear fruit. Billions of dollars and millions of lives will be affected by this immense wager.

There is reason for guarded, but not unbridled, optimism. As physicians and clinical investigators, we remain in equipoise about these experimental therapies. We are not in equipoise about clinical trials, however: we believe that best medical practice in the treatment of people with AD and other dementias includes discussion of possible clinical trial enrollment. We can empower our patients and their families to participate in the search for newer and better treatments. This heretofore progressive and fatal illness may become a chronic illness before too long; perhaps we can even do better than that. Along the way, we may also have to hark back to the basics: provide excellent care to those who suffer with this devastating illness, and therefore increase the likelihood of connecting motivated patients to clinical trials.

References

1. Rutten BP, Steinbusch HW, Korr H, et al. Antioxidants and Alzheimer's disease: from bench to bedside (and back again). Curr Opin Clin Nutr Metab Care 2002;5(6):645–651.

2. Birks J, Flicker L. Selegiline for Alzheimer's disease. Cochrane Database Syst Rev 2003;(1):CD000442.

3. Sano M, Ernesto C, Thomas RG, et al. A controlled trial of selegiline, alpha-tocopherol, or both as treatment for Alzheimer's disease. The Alzheimer's Disease Cooperative Study. N Engl J Med 1997;336(17):1216–1222.

4. Petersen RC, Thomas RG, Grundman M, et al. Vitamin E and donepezil for the treatment of mild cognitive impairment. N Engl J Med 2005;352(23):2379–2388.

5. Schneider LS, DeKosky ST, Farlow MR, et al. A randomized, double-blind, placebo-controlled trial of two doses of ginkgo biloba extract in dementia of the Alzheimer's type. Curr Alzheimer Res 2005;2(5):541–551.

6. DeKosky ST, Williamson JD, Fitzpatrick AL, et al. Ginkgo biloba for prevention of dementia. JAMA 2008;300(19):2253–2262.

7. Aisen PS, Davis KL, Berg JD, et al. A randomized controlled trial of prednisone in Alzheimer's disease. Alsheimer's Disease Cooperative Study. Neurology 2000;54:588–593.

8. Aisen PS, Schafer K, Gundman M, et al. Results of a multicenter trial of rofecoxib and naproxen in Alzheimer's disease. Neurobiology of Aging 2002;24:S429.

9. Breitner J, Buckholtz N, Molchan S, et al. Cognitive function over time in the Alzheimer's Disease Anti-inflammatory Prevention Trial (ADAPT). Arch Neurol 2008;65(7):869–905.

10. Fritze J, Walden J. Clinical findings with nimodipine in dementia: test of the calcium hypothesis. J Neural Transmission Suppl 1995;46:439–453.

11. Lopez-Arrieta JM, Birks J. Nimodipine for primary degenerative, mixed and vascular dementia. Cochrane Database Syst Rev 2002;(3):CD000147.

12. www.memorypharma.com

13. Tuszynski MH, Thal L, Pay M, et al. A phase 1 clinical trial of nerve growth factor gene therapy for Alzheimer disease. Nat Med 2005;11(5):551–555.

14. www.ceregene.com/press_050207.asp

15. Panisset M, Gauthier s. Moessler H, et al. Cerebrolysin in Alzheimer's disease: A randomized, double -blind, placebo-controlled trial with a neurotrophic agent. J Neural Transmission 2002;109(7–8):1089–1104.

16. Grundman M, Capparelli E, Kim HT, et al. A multicenter, randomized, placebo controlled, multiple-dose, safety and pharmacokinetic study of AIT-082 (neotrofin) in mild Alzheimer's disease patients. Life Sciences 2003;73(5):539–553.

17. Muresanu DF, Rainer M, Moessler H. Improved global funcion and activites of daily living inpatients with AD: A placebo-controlled clinical study with the neurotrophic agent Cerebrolysin. J Neural Transmission 2002;62(Suppl):177–185.

18. Simpkins JW, Singh M, Bishop J. The potential role for estrogen replacement therapy in the treatment of the cognitive decline and neurodegeneration associated with Alzheimer's disease. Neurobiology of Aging 1994;15(Suppl 2): S195–S197.

19. Paganini-Hill A, Henderson VW. Estrogen deficiency and risk of Alzheimer's disease in women. Am J Epidemiol 1994;140:256–261.

20. Asthana S, Baker LD, Craft S, et al. High-dose estradiol improves cognition for women with AD: Results of a randomized study. Neurology 2001;57:605–612.

21. Fillit H, Weinreb H, Cholst I, et al. Observations in a preliminary open trial of estradioltherapyforseniledementia-Alzheimer'stype.Psychoneuroendocrinology 1986;11:337–345.

22. Honjo H, Ogino Y, Naitoh K, et al. In vivo effects by estrone sulfate on the central nervous system-senile dementia (Alzheimer's type). J Steroid Biochem 1989;34:521–525.

23. Henderson VW, Paganini-Hill A, Miller BL, et al. Estrogen for Alzheimer's disease in women; Randomized, double-blind, placebo-controlled trial. Neurology 2000;54:295–301.

24. Mulnard RA, Cotman CW, Kawas C, et al. Estrogen replacement therapy for treatment of mild to moderate Alzheimer disease: A randomized controlled trial. Alzheimer's Disease Cooperative Study. JAMA 2000;283:1007–1015.

25. Shumaker SA, Legault C, Rapp Sr, et al. Estrogen plus progestin and the incidence of dementia and mild cognitive impairment in postmenopausal women: The Women's Health Initiative Memory Study. A randomized controlled trial. JAMA 2003;289:2651–2662.

Index

Note: Page numbers in *italics* refer to figures and tables.

247

LaVergne, TN USA
14 October 2010
200703LV00006B/1/P